THE LEAD DEBATE

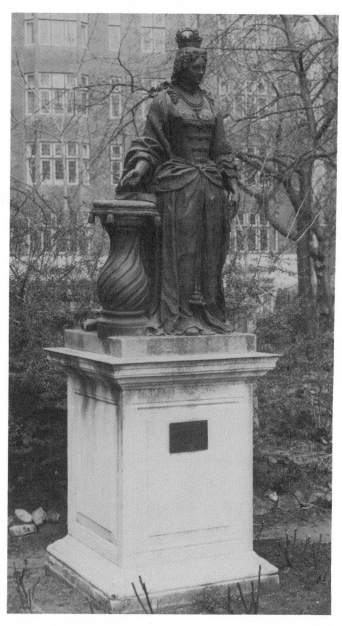

A lead statue of the Queen in Queen Square, London. (photograph copyright The Institute of Child Health/The Hospital for Sick Children, London)

The Lead Debate:

The Environment, Toxicology and Child Health

Edited by RICHARD LANSDOWN, PhD, FBPsS,
and
WILLIAM YULE, PhD, FBPsS

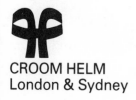

CROOM HELM
London & Sydney

© 1986 Richard Lansdown and William Yule
Croom Helm Ltd, Provident House, Burrell Row,
Beckenham, Kent BR3 1AT
Croom Helm Australia Pty Ltd, Suite 4, 6th Floor,
64-76 Kippax Street, Surry Hills, NSW 2010, Australia

British Library Cataloguing in Publication Data

The Lead debate: the environment, toxicology
 and child health.
 1. Lead-poisoning in children   2. Lead —
 Environmental aspects
 I. Lansdown, Richard   II. Yule, William
 613'.1   RA1231.L4
 ISBN 0-7099-1653-1
 ISBN 0-7099-1654-X Pbk

Typeset by Leaper & Gard Ltd, Bristol
Printed and bound in Great Britain by Mackays of Chatham Ltd, Kent

CONTENTS

ACKNOWLEDGEMENTS

We thank the following for kind permission to reproduce photographs, figures and tables as follows:

Frontispiece The Hospital for Sick Children, London
Chapter 3 Tables 3.1, 3.2, 3.3 World Bureau of Metal Statistics
Table 3.4 Paintmakers Association of Great Britain
Table 3.5 and Figures 3.1, 3.2, 3.3 The Lead Development Association
Chapter 6 Figures 6.1, 6.3, 6.5, 6.13 Her Majesty's Stationery Office
Table 6.1 and Figure 6.2 The National Institute of Enironmental Medicine, Stockholm
Figures 6.6, 6.8, 6.10, 6.12 John Wiley & Sons Ltd
Figures 6.7, 6.11 P.B. Hammond, R.L. Bornschein, P. Succop and C.S. Clark
Table 6.2 *Developmental Medicine & Child Neurology*
Chapter 8 Figure 8.1 American Chemical Society
Figure 8.2 A.C. Chamberlain
Figure 8.3 Commission of European Committees
Chapter 11 Figure 11.1 US Government Printing Office
Chapter 17 Figure 17.1 *New England Journal of Medicine*
Figure 17.2 John Wiley & Sons Ltd

FOREWORD

The Working party on Lead, of which Drs Yule and Lansdown were distinguished expert members and of which I was Chairman, was set up by the Department of Health and Social Security in November 1978 'To review the overall effects on health of environmental lead from all sources and, in particular, its effects on the health and development of children and to assess the contribution lead in petrol makes to the body burden.' The Report of the Working Party (HMSO, 1980) opens thus:

> Lead and its compounds are potentially toxic; the element has no known physiological functions; it is widely distributed in nature and as a result of man's activities. The gross effects which it can have on health have been recognised for many years and there are now relatively few cases of frank lead poisoning in this country. However, reports in recent years have suggested that there could be ill effects from exposure to lead in amounts which are too small to cause the classical signs and symptoms of lead poisoning.

It might have seemed to some that the burden laid upon the Working Party was not especially heavy but its task was formidable and involved the scrutiny of nearly 3000 publications of varied worth. There are many sources of lead among which are water, food, air and soil, as well as paint, cosmetics and medicines; the width of the range of indices of body burden among people sharing similar environmental circumstances suggests that there is no simple rule by the use of which one can attribute with certainty the roles played by individual sources. 'Behaviour' and 'intelligence' are difficult to define and are linked closely with social, genetic and physical factors; it must be accepted that, in many cases, it is impossible to attribute suspected deviations from accepted 'normal' values to environmental contamination yet the effort has to be made by the use of scrupulously fair and properly validated techniques.

The introduction to the Report states that 'Independent experts actively engaged in the fields of clinical paediatrics, pathology, child psychiatry, psychology, epidemiology and the environmental sciences were appointed'. Such was the complexity of the topic and the disparity of the various disciplines involved in assessment that much time had to be spent during which the experts in each discipline instructed their colleagues in the techniques which they employed in their individual approaches to the problems posed. The Working Party made its assessment and its 22 recommendations in the light of the information available but the Report, by its very nature, could not contain details more than that needed to justify its recommendations. The 'debate' goes on and this book, unhindered by stringent limits on its length, seeks to fill technical gaps and to help the sincere reader to make his own assessment, in the light of current work, of the role played by lead in the contemporary environment. Herein is detail in abundance and the legion references to published work are reminders that the subject is not new nor is it simple.

So, now read on — but with the care and academic humility which these many problems merit.

P.J. Lawther, CBE, MB, DSc, FRCP, FFOM,
Emeritus Professor of Environmental and Preventive Medicine,
St Bartholomew's Hospital, London

PREFACE

As anyone who is acquainted with the topic of this book will be aware, lead is a topic that arouses passions well beyond that normally encountered in scientific discourse. We have, at times, been the centre of debate and our work has been both heavily criticised and highly acclaimed. In this book we have tried to ensure that the picture is presented as we see it, in all its complexity, with no oversimplified conclusions.

We have tried, moreover, to compile a book which has something to offer both to the specialist in one of the many disciplines concerned with lead and children and to the more general reader. In order to achieve these aims we have included some chapters of an introductory nature and others written with the more informed reader in mind.

We are most grateful to all our contributors, especially Professor Pat Lawther, who not only wrote the Foreword but also made detailed comments on much of the book's content.

Richard Lansdown
William Yule

LIST OF CONTRIBUTORS

Philippe Grandjean, Department of Environmental Medicine, Institute of Community Health, Odense University, J.B. Winsløws Vej 19, DK-5000 Odense C, Denmark.

Janet Hunter, formerly Department of Psychology, Institute of Psychiatry. Now at Inner London Education Authority, Research and Statistics Department, County Hall, London SE1 7PB.

Richard Lansdown, Chief Psychologist, Department of Psychological Medicine, The Hospitals for Sick Children, Great Ormond Street, London WC1N 3JH.

Michael R. Moore, Department of Medicine, University of Glasgow, Glasgow, Scotland.

Marjorie Smith, Institute of Child Health, University of London, 30 Guilford Street, London WC1N 1EH.

Marie Anne Urbanowicz, Department of Clinical Psychology, Institute of Psychiatry, de Crespigny Park, London SE5 8AF.

Gerhard Winneke, Med. Institut für Umwelthygiene an der Universität Düsseldorf, Gurlittstrasse 53,4000 Düsseldorf 1, Federal Republic of Germany.

William Yule, Reader in Applied Child Psychology, Department of Clinical Psychology, Institute of Psychiatry, de Crespigny Park, London SE5 8AF.

PART ONE

BACKGROUND

1 WHAT IS LEAD?

Marjorie Smith

Lead is a metal. Technically metals are the large group of elements which form positive ions in solution. Within this group there are several different methods of subdividing or grouping metals. Chemists subdivide them by their chemical properties, physicists by their physical properties, and engineers by their mechanical or structural properties. Originally the group of known (or recognised) metals was divided into the precious or noble metals, which were gold and silver, and the base metals such as lead, copper and iron. More recently lead would be described as a heavy metal. To a metallurgist this would mean that lead, along with metals such as gold, iron, aluminium and cobalt, had an atomic weight greater than that of sodium, and that it formed soaps on reaction with fatty acids. By this classification the so-called alkali metals, such as potassium, lithium and sodium are light metals. Sometimes lead is described as a heavy metal because of its density. In this case the newer, less dense metals such as aluminium would be called light metals.

In appearance lead originally has a shiny silver lustre, but it quickly weathers to take on the more familiar dull grey-bluish colour. It is unique among common metals in being very soft and malleable, but at the same time having virtually no elasticity, and little mechanical strength. Since it is a heavy dense metal this lack of mechanical strength and softness means that lead has a tendency to flow, or creep, under its own weight. It is resistant to corrosion because of the film of lead carbonate which forms on the surface as a result of the reaction between lead and air. It is this protective film which gives lead its dull grey appearance, in contrast to the shiny appearance of freshly cut lead.

In the periodic table of elements the chemical symbol for lead is Pb, from the Latin name for lead, which was plumbum. Elements can be described by their atomic weight. This is the mass of the atom, on a scale which used to be based on the weight equivalent per atom of hydrogen, but is now based on equivalence to atoms of the isotope carbon-12, which is assigned an atomic weight of twelve. Most atomic weights are not whole numbers because an

3

element is usually made up of two or more isotopes. There are different 'versions' of the atom, with the same charge on the nucleus, and the same chemical and physical properties, but with a different atomic weight. The naturally occuring isotopes of lead have atomic weights of 204, 206, 207, 208 and 210, and calculated from the assumed natural isotopic combination, this gives lead an atomic weight of 207.2. Three of the stable isotopes, lead 206, 207 and 208, are the end products of the radioactive decay of uranium, actinium and thorium. Because of this lead ores which were deposited in different places during different geological periods show distinct isotopic mixtures. This means that the lead obtained from the important historic mining areas of Greece, Spain and Britain can be distinguished on the basis of its isotopic combination.

Lead is one of the seven metals which have been known to man since prehistoric times. Unlike gold, silver and copper, lead is not found in nature in its metallic state. Thus all lead has to be obtained from its ores. An ore is a compound or mineral occurring naturally in the earth's crust from which the metal can be extracted. The principal lead ore is galena (lead sulphide) which is found as a shiny black metallic-looking stone. Cerussite (lead carbonate), anglesite (lead sulphate) and less commonly crocoite and wulfenite are other ores which are weathered products of galena, and are generally found nearer the surface. Approximately 0.002 per cent of the earth's crust is lead, localised into deposits sufficiently rich to justify mining (Lead Development Association, 1974). Lead ores are widely distributed with deposits found in all five continents.

Forms of Lead

Lead is present in the world today in a large number of different guises. However, these may be simply divided into lead in metallic form, and lead in the form of chemical compounds. The properties and behaviour of lead in its different forms may be very different. In metallic form lead may be further subdivided into unalloyed lead, and lead alloys. Unalloyed lead is lead with no intentional additions of other metals. Although lead of a high degree of purity can be made, it will always contain some impurities, but in unalloyed lead these are unintentional. 'Pure' lead has a melting point of 327°C, which is lower than the melting points of other common metals with the exception of tin.

Lead alloys are formed by the controlled addition of other metals to lead. The purpose of this is selectively to change the metal's properties. For example alloys of lead can be created with greater hardness and increased mechanical strength, without changing the resistance to corrosion, or alternatively if corrosion resistance is of importance, an alloy of lead and copper will, under certain conditions of exposure, give greater corrosion resistance. The properties of alloys are different from those of either of their 'parent' metals. For example if a lead and tin alloy is heated, the temperature at which the alloy starts to solidify on cooling, is lower than that for either lead or tin. Even very small additions of other metals may significantly change the properties of lead. Adding less than 0.1 per cent of tellurium to lead will improve the mechanical strength of lead significantly.

In metallic form lead is virtually insoluble in pure water. However, in the presence of air, lead is attacked by pure (distilled) water, and forms lead hydroxide which is appreciably soluble. This action is due partly to dissolved oxygen, and partly to free carbonic acid, and so it can occur only in the presence of air. Soft water (or rain water) does not contain salts and is therefore a pure water, and its action is plumbosolvent, that is, it dissolves lead. Hard water contains salts which produce a carbonate film on the surface of the lead, and protect it from further attack, and thus lead is much less soluble in hard water. One of the properties of lead which has proved useful is its insolubility in (cold) concentrated sulphuric acid. The solubility of lead compounds in water varies widely; some such as lead acetate and lead nitrate are quite soluble in water, whereas most compounds, for example lead chromate and the lead oxides, are largely insoluble in water.

Lead compounds may be divided into organic and inorganic compounds. Organic lead compounds are those which contain carbon and hydrogen. Organic lead compounds which contain at least one lead-carbon bond are known as organolead compounds. The best-known examples of these are tetra-ethyl lead, and tetramethyl lead, which have been widely used as anti-knock additives to petrol. Organic (or organo-) lead compounds can be converted into inorganic compounds. The high pressure, and high temperature necessary for combustion within a car engine (and the presence of bromine compounds as scavengers in the petrol) converts the organolead present in the petrol into an inorganic form which is then largely discharged in the exhaust fumes. The discharged lead will be mostly in the form of small particles (i.e. particles of less than 10 µm in size) and some of these may be attached to particles of carbon in the exhaust. Some of the lead particles will remain in the engine or exhaust system of the car, until a sudden acceleration causes a burst of exhaust gases and this will dislodge some of these larger particles. The relevance of particle size is that the size and shape of the particle governs its dispersal. The smaller the particle the further it will travel. Large particles will settle almost immediately, but smaller particles may be carried some distance by the wind. Similarly within the human body, the size of respired or ingested lead particles is of crucial importance in determining the rate and degree of absorption.

Man has mined and used lead for many thousands of years, and this has resulted in an accumulation of environmental lead. Unlike many other substances produced or used by man, and particularly other pollutants, lead has a long environmental residence time. In practice this means that it is difficult to get rid of. Once lead has been taken out of the earth there is no way of disposing of it, and no inert or innocuous form into which it can be converted in the environment. To compare the environmental residence time of two pollutants produced by cars: 50 per cent of a one metre column of carbon monoxide in contact with soil will remain in half an hour, whereas 90 per cent of the lead in upper layers of moorland soil will still be there between 70 and 200 years later (DHSS, 1980).

References

DHSS (1980) *Lead and Health: The Report of a DHSS Working Party on Lead in the Environment.* (The Lawther Report). HMSO, London.
Lead Development Association (1974) *Technical notes on Lead: Production Properties and Uses.* Lead Development Association, London.

2 LEAD IN HISTORY

Marjorie Smith

Earliest Knowledge of Lead

The first metals used by man were almost certainly those such as gold, which are found in their metallic state. The bright shiny pebble-like objects which might be found in the beds of rivers would attract attention and were probably first collected as curiosities before man discovered that the material could be made into useful or decorative objects. Some time later man would have discovered that by heating native gold or copper it became more workable.

At a later stage man learned to produce metals from their ore. There is dispute about which metal was the first to be obtained from its ore, with some authorities maintaining that it was copper. Krysko (1979) puts forward a convincing case for lead being the first metal to be smelted. He points out that lead was the easiest metal to smelt, requiring only a modest temperature which could easily be achieved on a camp fire, compared with a temperature of over 1000°C required to smelt copper. Krysko pictures man experimenting some ten thousand years ago, to discover the reactions of different types of stones to heating, and discovering that the shiny brittle stone that was galena, could be transformed by fire into a malleable and different form. Since ancient man had experience with other metals he would have recognised this as a metal with properties, such as its softness and malleability, which were different from the metals he already knew. Since lead is not found in its metallic state the appearance of metallic lead is evidence that man had learnt to smelt ore to produce the metal. Small beads of metallic lead have been found with gold and copper objects dating from 7000-6500 BC, in excavations on the central Anatolian Plain. This is some two thousand years earlier than the evidence of the first copper smelting (Krysko, 1979).

Lead in the Ancient World

The history of lead is closely bound to the history of silver, since galena ore also contains silver. Although silver is found in its native state, galena is by far the most abundant source. At the surface the silver content of galena ore may be precipitated as metallic silver, and it may have been this which led early man to experiment with the material in the layers beneath. Much of the mining of lead ores throughout history has been in order to obtain silver, with the lead obtained considered as a waste product of little or no value. In fact lead mines were often called silver mines.

In silver-containing lead ores the silver is obtained by heating the molten lead for longer, causing it to change into litharge (lead oxide) and silver. Litharge, which is a yellow glaze, has been found on glazed ceramics dating from 5000 BC (Krysko, 1979). Quantities of litharge have been found round ancient mines which provides evidence that the mines were worked for their silver content, and not for the lead. The process of cupellation by which lead-silver alloy is separated into silver and lead was described as a 'very old' process on cuneiform tablets found at Assur, and dating from about the second millenium BC (Krysko, 1979).

The Egyptians, Phoenecians and Hebrews all used lead, but not in large quantities or for large objects. Lucas and Harris (1962) describe the ancient Egyptians using metallic lead for small human and animal figurines; sinkers for fishing nets; rings, beads and other small ornaments; model dishes and trays; vessels, tanks and plugs. In addition lead was added to bronze in quantities up to 20 per cent, to produce what was later described by Pliny as 'statue metal'. The effect of adding lead to bronze significantly reduces the melting point and makes casting easier. Galena, ground to a powder, was used as eye paint in ancient Egypt as early as Badarian times, and several oxides were used as pigments for decorations or for writing.

The oldest known decorative man-made lead object is a small carved figure of a woman dating from about 4000 BC, discovered in the temple of Osiris in Egypt. Most other decorative objects dating from the third and second millenia BC are of this type, small human or animal figurines, probably used as votive objects, and produced in quantity by casting in a mould.

Although the earliest knowledge of metallurgy probably originated in the middle and far East, by about 1500 BC this knowledge had spread along the trade routes and from this time leaden objects or articles made from lead alloys have been found in many parts of the world. Two gilded lead pendants dating from about 1500 BC have been found in Ireland (Krysko, 1979).

The main uses of lead in the ancient world were for small decorative objects such as those described, and for a range of practical uses such as standard weights and sinkers, to which the softness and malleability of lead lent itself. Because of its low melting point lead was used as solder (usually as lead-tin alloy) for jointing other metals. Lead was also used in coinage, either in its pure form or as a lead alloy. In Assyria animal heads made out of lead were used as the most common form of exchange in the period 1400-1050 BC (Nriagu, 1983). Oxides or compounds of lead have been used in prehistoric times as cosmetics: in addition to the Egyptian use of galena as eye paint, in China and in classical Greece, white lead (ceruse) was used to whiten the face; for pigments, for glazes, and for glass. Lead has been used in glass for more than two and a half millenia. It has been used to increase the brilliance of glass and to make it easier to cut or engrave, and also to colour glass. Small objects made of brightly coloured opaque glass, dating from the fifteenth century BC, have been found all over the middle East.

Apart from artefacts and objects surviving from the prehistoric period there are many written references to lead, including several references in the Old Testament. In Ezekial there is a mention of lead, as well as silver, iron and tin, among the 'riches' which were traded in the fairs (*Ezekial*, 27:12). There are several mentions of the process of cupellation, and of lead as the 'dross' of the silver, but in Jeremiah there is a description of the process: 'The bellows are burned, the lead is consumed of the fire, the founder melteth in vain, for the wicked are not plucked away. Reprobate silver shall men call them, because the Lord hath rejected them' (*Jeremiah*, 6:29-30). In the book of Job there is a reference to the use of lead tablets for writing on, in the verse preceding the lines made famous by the air from Handel's *Messiah*:

Oh that my words were now written! oh that they were printed in a book! That they were graven with an iron pen and lead in the rock forever!
For I know that my redeemer liveth, and that he shall stand at the latter day upon the earth. (*Job*, 19:23-25).

Messages inscribed on metal plates, some of which were lead, have been used since 3000 BC as a way of making a permanent record.

These heavy metal plates were sometimes buried in the foundations of temples (Krysko, 1979).

References to lead in ancient literature are complicated by the
lack of distinction between lead and tin. Pliny (cited by Nriagu,
1983) demonstrated this confusion by describing two kinds of
'lead': plumbum nigrum (black lead) which was lead, and plumbum album (white lead) which was tin.

The Roman Period

Until the Roman era the amount of lead used was small in
comparison to the usage of other metals, and lead was a very
unimportant metal. However the Romans changed that. In the
Roman era, as later, metals meant wealth. The spread of the
Roman empire, and therefore the invasion of Britain, was partly
due to the need for metals.

It is probable that lead was mined on a small scale in Britain
before the Roman conquest. Certainly Caesar's expedition to
Britain was prompted by a knowledge of the existence of lead in
Britain, and by the belief that there was a great mineral wealth in
the country (Pulsifer, 1888). Since the galena found in Britain
contains very little silver, although this would have been extracted,
it is clear that the Romans were motivated by their need for lead. It
is known that the lead mines of the Mendips were being worked by
49 AD, which is only six years after the Roman conquest (Tylecote, 1976). Mines were worked in Northumberland, Cumberland,
Yorkshire, Derbyshire, Shropshire, in the Mendips in Somerset, in
Devon and Cornwall and in Wales. In almost every area in Britain
where lead mining has been carried out in more recent times, the
signs of ancient mining can be found. Pulsifer (1888) suggests that
the choice of York as the northern capital of Britain, may have
been due to its proximity to the lead mining areas on Alston Moor
and South Yorkshire. Describing the extensive Roman mining
operations which probably lasted over three centuries, Pulsifer says
'The tribute paid to Britain by the Roman Empire consisted principally of lead'.

Since Roman times ingots of lead, called pigs, have been
marked with the maker's name, or the name of the mine from
which the ore was produced, and often with other information as
well. Several lead pigs from Roman times have been found in

Britain. One, found in Hampshire in 1783 and now in the British Museum, bears the inscription: NERON.AVG.EX KIAN III COS BRIT, and on the reverse: EX ARGENT. CNPASCI. This shows that it was produced in the time of Nero (about AD 60) from the mines of Kiani in Wales, and that it is free of silver. The Romans could desilverise lead to a purity of 99.95 per cent.

Much of the lead produced from British mines was used in Britain, but some was exported to France and to Rome. The main use of lead in the Roman period was for sanitary engineering — that is for the elaborate systems of piping and cisterns which supplied water to towns and houses throughout the Roman Empire. In the Roman era cisterns and pipes were made from cast lead sheet. The casting techniques used by the Romans remained largely unchanged until the late eighteenth century, when lead sheet began to be produced by rolling and milling (Rowe, 1983). The technique involved pouring molten lead into a shallow flat bed made of sand or a mixture of dried clay and sand. The molten lead cooled to form a thin sheet. The dried clay and sand moulds were sometimes decorated with embossed ornamentation, or with the maker's name. The extravagant use of lead in Roman times is demonstrated by the fact that the Roman Baths in Bath are lined with lead weighing 40 lb to the square foot.

Lead sheets of standard size were used to make pipes, which in the Roman empire were standardised to a length of ten Roman feet, and to one of ten standard diameters. There were two ways of making pipes. Probably the most commonly used method was to wrap the lead sheet around a cylindrical core of the correct diameter, abutting the edges of the lead sheet. Hot lead was then poured onto these edges, melting them together and forming a ridged, welded joint. A second method, essentially similar, was described by Pliny (cited by Krysko, 1979), in which the joint was made by soldering with a lead-tin alloy. This produced a round pipe without a longitudinal ridge. That the Romans were successful pipe makers is evidenced by the fact that some welded Roman pipes, such as those in the Roman Baths in Bath, have been in use almost continuously since Roman times. The welding method of pipe manufacture was used until the mid-eighteenth century when casting became the most common method of pipe production (Rowe, 1983).

The Romans had other uses for lead. Lead sheet was used for roofing, and for covering and protecting the keels of ships. It was also used to make ships' anchors, and for weights of all kinds. Domestically lead was used in a variety of cooking pots, utensils, and for plates and drinking vessels. Cooking pots made of bronze were often lined with lead to stop the taste of copper contaminating the contents. Much of the domestic ware was made of pewter (called poor man's metal) which in Roman times was 50 per cent lead and 50 per cent tin. Other domestic uses included ornaments and jewellery, cosmetics and some medicinal remedies. Several curious properties were ascribed to lead in Roman times. The emperor Nero is reported by Pliny, to have worn a breastplate made of lead to help him sing (Pulsifer, 1888).

As in prehistoric times lead compounds were used as pigments for colouring and in glass. Another use which persisted since ancient times was the use of lead for burials. Since the earliest times lead urns had been used for preserving the ashes or vital organs of the dead. In Roman times with the spread of Christianity and the burial of the dead, lead was used to make or line sarcophagi. These were usually made very simply by folding the edges of a lead sheet up to make a rectangular box, with the lid made in the same manner. Later decorated sarcophagi were produced by means of patterns or emblems embossed from the casting moulds.

With the decline of the economy of the Roman empire before its downfall, lead began to be used in coinage to reduce the amount of silver it contained. Another use of lead during the decline of the empire was to make tokens called tesserae. These lead tokens, stamped or embossed with a mark which identified their purpose, were issued to the masses of unemployed. They were used, among other things, to control the distribution of grain, to gain entrance to the Colosseum, to entitle the holder to free wine, or even to gain free entrance to one of the Imperial brothels (Krysko, 1979).

With the fall of the Roman civilisation and with it the desire for cleanliness, the need for lead declined. What little lead was used was probably salvaged from the large quantities of Roman lead lying around, and it was not until the early Middle Ages that lead began to be mined again in Britain.

The Middle Ages and the Renaissance

In the Middle Ages and until the Renaissance lead was a metal surrounded by superstition and prejudice. Even in the early seventeenth century Le Febvre writing in his *Compendious Body of Chymistry* says 'Lead is the vilest and most abject of metals'. The long use of lead as a mortuary metal, and therefore its association with death, may have accounted for some of this prejudice, but also the attentions of alchemists led to associations with cults, magic and evil (Krysko, 1979). Although the alchemists regarded lead as the ancestor or father of all metals (as did the ancient Chinese, Egyptian and Indian cultures) it was at the same time regarded as the least of them. Much of the scientific effort and experimentation of the Middle Ages was directed towards the attempt to transmute base lead into gold.

Despite the prejudice against lead, with the gradual return of the desire for cleanliness there was a need for lead, and many of the old Roman mines were opened and reworked. In the twelfth and thirteenth centuries the chief lead-producing centres in England were Cumberland, Yorkshire, Northumberland, Derbyshire, the Mendips and Shropshire. As in Roman times the main practical uses of lead were for roofing and piping. People went considerable distances to buy lead. In 1222 there is a record of the Major of Winchester travelling to Boston fair in Lincolnshire to buy lead for roofing Winchester Castle (Cordero and Tarry, 1960). In 1285 lead pipes were laid in Cheapside in the City of London to supply the city with water brought from Paddington.

Lead has been used in warfare since ancient times. It was originally used to make sling bullets. In the early middle ages the crusaders used molten lead to pour onto the heads of enemies threatening to invade their castles. Later in the fourteenth century with the invention of the musket, there was a demand for lead for bullets. Lead shot was made either by casting to make large bullets, or later in the mid-seventeenth century small shot was made by dropping lead through a sieve into water (Rowe, 1983).

In the Middle Ages much of the domestic ware of the merchant classes was made of pewter, containing up to 60 per cent lead. From 1450 onwards lead was used in place of money when coinage was in short supply, in glass, and in strips to hold pieces of coloured glass together in church and cathedral windows. A plumber in the Middle Ages, and until relatively recently, was a worker in lead, so as well as piping he performed other skills, such as roofing, involving lead. The church records of East Dereham in Norfolk contain a note dated 1468 which says 'Paid William, the plumber, for leading the new font, 2s 6d.' (Pulsifer, 1888).

In Tudor times Cardinal Wolsey had more than eight miles of lead pipe laid in order to supply water to Hampton Court palace (Pulsifer, 1888). In Elizabethan England mining of all sorts expanded, and lead was produced for the home market as well as for export. By the seventeenth century half the exports of Britain were lead or tin, so it is probable that Britain supplied much of the continental requirements. The industrial activities involved in producing lead as well as iron, and the new manufacture of glass, denuded many of the forests of England. Until the Elizabethan period lead had been extracted from the ore in small bole furnaces, often known as 'bole-hills'. These primitive furnaces had a poor yield but were easy and cheap to operate as they could use almost any sort of dry fuel such as peat, coal or wood. They were usually sited on hill tops to make the most of the natural draught, and because the fumes killed the vegetation for miles around. In the Elizabethan period foot operated, bellows-blown furnaces, fuelled by wood, made the process much more efficient.

The advent of the large country house in the seventeenth century caused a renewed demand for lead for roofing, piping, and for a new use, statuary. This demand was probably inspired in part, by the building, between 1668 and 1671, of Louis XIV's chateau at Versailles. One hundred thousand square metres of English lead were used to cover the roof. For the first time lead was extensively used for large-scale ornamentation, in the many statues and fountains which were originally gilded, and which still decorate the gardens at Versailles.

Until the seventeenth century the skills necessary to make large structures in lead were not widely known, although there are isolated examples of these skills from two centuries earlier. Lead has a tendency to creep under its own weight, and so any large object made of lead would have developed cracks and eventually collapsed. Alloying lead is one way of avoiding creep, but from the 1600s there is evidence that techniques of preventing creep by providing a rigid supporting framework were becoming known, and this enabled large constructions to be made in lead. Since lead cannot be X-rayed the evidence of these skills becomes apparent only when statues need repair. A supporting framework was revealed when a lead fountain which was erected in 1408 was severely damaged by fire (Krysko, 1979). However, it is clear that these skills, often in combination with alloying techniques were widely known by the seventeenth century, and until the end of the eighteenth century lead was a very fashionable material for a wide variety of statuary and ornamentation. Monuments and statues in lead dating from this time can be seen in many cities and towns, as well as decorating private gardens.

The Industrial Revolution

In the last half of the eighteenth century scientific inventions and the rising population increased the rate of industrial change. Many of the modern uses of lead, described in the next chapter, were invented during this period. The invention by John Roebuck in 1746 of the lead chamber process for the manufacture of sulphuric acid, is regarded by chemists as one of the most significant developments of the Industrial Revolution (Rowe, 1983). A better method of producing lead shot came with the invention of the shot tower by William Watts, who was a plumber in Bristol, in 1782. Rowe (1983) tells two versions of the story of how Watts came to discover the process. The first version tells of the inebriated Watts falling into a stupor at the foot of the tower of St Mary, Redcliffe. He dreamed that the church caught fire, and that the lead from the roof melted and fell to the ground where it landed in pools of water and formed perfectly spherical shot. The alternative version is perhaps a better story. This relates that the drunken Watts dreamed that his wife was standing on the church tower pouring molten lead on him through the holes in a rusty frying pan. Whether these unlikely stories are true or not, Watts and his wife obtained permission to use the church tower to experiment, and found that the process did actually work as his drunken dreams had apparently predicted. Watts took out a patent on this process in 1782, and in 1785 he adapted a house in Bristol to construct the first shot tower.

The first lead storage battery was made in 1859 when Gaston Plante used two lead plates in a bath of acid. His design was later modified by a colleague to create a battery essentially similar to those in use today. The use of lead as electrodes in accumulators for the storage of electricity created a new demand for lead.

Lead Poisoning and the Knowledge of Lead Toxicity

It is probable that the toxic effects of lead have been known for almost as long as lead itself, but descriptions of lead poisoning are uncommon in ancient literature. The Greeks and Romans undoubtedly knew about lead toxicity, and they were familiar with the symptoms of lead poisoning. Given the prodigious use of lead in Roman times it is likely that poisoning from occupational and non-occupational exposure to lead was a relatively common hazard. Both Pliny and Vitruvius warn of the toxic effect of the fumes given off by heated lead. Pliny writes, 'For medicinal purposes lead is melted in earthen vessels, ... whilst it is being melted the breathing passages should be protected ... otherwise the noxious and deadly vapour of the lead furnace is inhaled; it is harmful to dogs with special rapidity.' Pliny also says, 'red lead is a deadly poison and should not be used medicinally', and both Pliny and Celsus warn of the deadly nature of white lead (Waldron, 1973).

This knowledge did not stop the Greeks and Romans exposing themselves to considerable quantities of lead from water, wine, cooking pots and food, and medicines. Since sugar was not available the Romans used reduced raw grape juice, called sapa or defrutum according to the degree of boiling down, as a sweetening agent. Columella and Pliny both specifically recommend that this should be made in a leaden pot. Pliny (quoted by Gilfillan, 1965) says, 'Leaden and not bronze pots should be used.' To reduce the sweetening syrup to a half or a third of its original volume as was recommended, would have necessitated boiling for some time, and this would have resulted in the sapa or defrutum being contaminated with considerable quantities of lead. Sapa and defrutum were widely added to food including meat and fish dishes, and sapa was also added to poor wine to sweeten it, and was used to preserve fruit. Lead inhibits enzyme activity, and this meant that the lead-containing sapa had the advantage (from the Roman point of view) of preserving fruit and inhibiting fermentation, and of preventing wine from souring. Gilfillan (1965) claims that the Romans added lead to their wine in up to fourteen different ways, including boiling the must before fermenting it, and warming wine in a lead-lined vessel before serving it. Gilfillan (1965) has estimated that wine sweetened with sapa prepared in leaden pots could contain up to 1000mg/l lead. Even a teaspoonful of this per day could have caused chronic lead poisoning. The toxic effects of adding sapa to improve the taste of poor wine were recognised. Pliny wrote of the adulterated wines, 'from the excessive use of such wines arise dangling ... paralytic hands', and Dioscorides noted that such wine was 'most hurtful to the nerves' (both quoted by Waldron, 1973).

The effects of metallic lead in the form of water pipes were also tentatively recognised by Vitruvius, who wrote:

> water is much more wholesome from earthernware than from lead pipes. For it seems to be made injurious by lead because cerusse is produced by it; and this is said to be harmful to the human body. Thus if what is produced by anything is injurious, it is not doubtful but that the thing is unwholesome in itself.
>
> We may take example by the workers in lead who have complexions affected by pallor. For when, in casting, the lead receives the current of air, the fumes from it occupy the members of the body and rob the limbs of the virtues of the blood. Therefore it seems that water should not be brought in lead pipes if we desire to have it wholesome. (quoted by Waldron, 1973)

Other than this rather lateral reference to lead workers by Vitruvius, there is very little literary evidence of the dangers of occupational exposure in Roman times, although with large quantities of lead being produced and worked this must have affected a considerable number of the population. Galena was the principal ore mined in ancient times, and this is relatively non-toxic. However the process of smelting, and of cupellation to separate out the silver, as would have happened at the great Athenian silver mine at Laurium, would have caused toxic fumes to be given off. McCord (1953) quotes Durant as saying, 'Laurium pays the price of the wealth it produces, ... plants and men wither and die from the furnace fumes, and the vicinity of the works becomes a scene of dusty desolation.' The majority of references to occupational exposure are from non-medical writers, and this suggests that physicians were little concerned with the diseases and ills which affected working people.

The earliest clinical description of lead poisoning has often been attributed to Hippocrates in 370 BC. In the third book of *Epidemics* Hippocrates describes symptoms of colic and constipation as one of the frequent and dangerous endemic disorders, and although the description could be one of plumbism, it is not sufficiently specific to tell whether this is so, and no mention is made of lead as the cause (Waldron, 1973). The credit for the first undoubted account must go to Nikander, who, in the second century BC, gave a clear account of the poisonous effects of litharge and cerusse. Nikander was a Greek poet and physician who described in verse in his Alexipharmac, the effects of poisons and their antidotes. His description of lead poisoning includes pallor, colic, paralysis and drooping limbs, occular disturbances and death (Major, 1945).

Although it is clear that the Romans knew about lead poisoning, it is difficult to judge how common it was. An epidemic of lead colic which, 'took its origin from regions in Italy, moreover in many other places in Roman territory, whence it spread like the contagion of a pestilential plague', was described by Paul of Aegina, a Greek physician of the seventh century, but he did not recognise the cause of this 'epidemic' (Major, 1945). Gilfillan (1965) has put forward the theory that the fall of the Roman empire was the result of lead poisoning. He suggests that the low birth rate and the high child mortality among the Roman aristocracy were caused by lead poisoning, and attributes the decline of the Roman civilisation to this 'aristothanasia'. As Waldron (1973) points out, the 'fall' of Rome was actually a very gradual process, and while lead may have been one negative influence, it was certainly not the only one.

Evidence, from the analysis of bones of the body lead burdens in ancient times is relatively sparse. Bone samples from the Romanised town of Cirencester were found to have lead levels very much higher than modern levels, and higher than samples from pre-Roman sites at Bath and Danebury, but this is not so for all samples of Roman bone analysed. Low lead levels have been found in bones from Verulamium, and it is suggested that these were from an impoverished group of native Britons. Levels comparable with modern ones have been found in bones from several Roman British sites. More recent results cited by Nriagu (1983) from the analysis of Roman and later bones, led to the conclusion that the lead burden of the Roman population was comparable with that found in bones dating from the Middle Ages.

One of the curious features of the history of lead is that knowledge of lead toxicity and the effects of lead have been periodically ignored and then (on occasions) rediscovered. Lead poisoning has been described as an 'aping disease' (McCord, 1954) because of the wide range of symptoms which it may produce, and the number of other diseases which it may imitate, and this may be one reason why the cause is often not recognised. It seems that the toxicity of lead compounds has been recognised more or less continuously, whereas the toxic effects associated with the use of metallic lead, perhaps because it appears so inert, are periodically forgotten. Lead acetate was known as 'inheritance powder', because of its known use as a poison. It was ground to make a sweet-tasting powder which was almost undetectable in food, and it had a long history as a poison used by those hoping to gain by the death of a close relative (Krysko, 1979).

Since Paul of Aegina described an epidemic of lead poisoning occurring in the seventh century, there have been other descriptions of similar epidemics. In 1616 Francois Citois who was born in Poitiers, in France, published an account of an epidemic characterised by symptoms of pallor, disturbances of the mind and of vision, insomnia, fainting, stomach pains, loss of appetite, nausea, vomiting, inflamed abdomen, convulsions and paralysis. This he called colica Pictonum, although after a later description by Dehaen in 1754 it became better known as Poitiers colic.

In 1738, John Huxham provided a clear description of similar symptoms said 'to infest the county of Devon, amongst the populace especially, and those who were not very elegant and careful in their diet'. These epidemics of what became known as Devonshire colic, occurred almost every autumn. Huxham noted that the symptoms were exacerbated by drinking beer or cider, and that children were not so severely affected as adults. These observations may have been accurate, but he was less accurate when he observed that 'this distemper was most violent when northerly winds prevailed' (Major, 1945). Some time later it was recognised that cider drinking was in some way related to the cause, but the real reason for these epidemics was not recognised for thirty years. In the case of Poitiers colic the cause was unrecognised for 150 years after the first description by Citois.

Another local epidemic occurred on French warships in the nineteenth century. At the time it was assumed that the disease was caused by a tropical miasma. In fact it was caused by lead poisoning from the water supply. At that time the dangers of scurvy were recognised, and so most fleets carried fruit or fruit juice. For economy the French fleet used vinegar or apple juice which was put in the water supply. This had the effect of making the water acidic and therefore plumbosolvent. The connecting pipes from the tanks to the ships were lead, and the water passing through these pipes picked up enough lead to contaminate the ships' entire water supply (Schadewaldt, 1967).

In the 1750s and 1760s there came a re-awakening to knowledge of the dangers of lead. This started in Europe with publications by Tronchin and Baker, but soon spread to America. In 1757 Tronchin published an essay in which he put forward the hypothesis that colica Pictonum or Poitiers colic, in Amsterdam, was caused by rain water which had passed over leaden roofs being kept for drinking purposes. He drew parallels between the observed effects of lead given for medicinal reasons, the ills suffered by miners of red lead, and the effects of wine which had been adulterated with litharge. Sir George Baker was more definite in solving the puzzle of Devonshire colic. In his paper read to the Royal College of Physicians in 1767, Baker reported that as a result of the observations of a doctor in Worcester, he had carried out some experiments. The doctor had observed a colic similar to Devonshire colic (which was not known in the cider-drinking counties of Hereford, Gloucester, and Worcester) on two occasions when cider was put into leaden cisterns, or made in a leaden press. Baker had observed that unlike the Herefordshire presses, cider presses in Devon were lead lined. He was able to show, by experimentation, that the Devon cider contained lead, and that this was the cause of the colic. This pronouncement brought condemnation from the clergy, members of the medical profession, and not surprisingly, from the mill owners.

The revival of the medical appreciation of lead toxicity in Europe may have been stimulated by information from Benjamin Franklin in America. Franklin was not medically qualified, but his experience and interest had given him insight into the dangers of lead. In 1724 while in England, Franklin worked as a printer's apprentice, and had observed that the practice of heating the lead type during cleaning resulted in what he called 'dangles'. In 1745 Franklin was the publisher (though not the author) of an essay on '*Dry Gripes*'. America had for some time been plagued with epidemics of the 'dry gripes'. These had been traced to rum drinking, and Franklin had observed that they were caused by the use of lead worms and still heads in the distillation process. Franklin and Baker knew each other, or at least corresponded, and in 1768 Baker says that his suspicions that lead might be the cause of Devonshire colic had been 'greatly confirmed by the authority of Dr Franklin of Philadelphia'. However Franklin never published on the subject of lead poisoning. In 1786 he wrote a long letter to a friend, following a conversation on the effects of lead. In the letter he sets out chronologically the development of his knowledge of lead toxicity, starting with his experience as a printer's apprentice. Franklin ends the letter by saying:

> This my dear Friend, is all I can at present recollect on the Subject. You will see by it, that the Opinion of the mischievious Effect from Lead is at least above Sixty Years old; and you will observe with Concern how long a useful Truth may be known and exist, before it is generally receiv'd and practic'd on. (quoted by McCord, 1953)

In 1840 Burton, a physician at St Thomas's Hospital in London, published a paper entitled *On the remarkable effect on human gums produced by the absorption of lead.* This paper described how Burton had noted that in lead-poisoned patients the edges of the gums 'were distinctly bordered by a narrow leaden-blue line, about one-twentieth part of an inch in width' (Major, 1945). This discovery of lead lines made the subsequent diagnosis of lead poisoning, in its many guises, a much easier one to make. It is interesting to note that in 1840 when Burton wrote his paper, acetate of lead was still being prescribed for medicinal reasons to patients in St Thomas's Hospital.

During the Industrial Revolution, with more people employed in factories and the increased use of lead in industrial processes, lead poisoning from occupational exposure increased. In 1767 Franklin obtained a listing of all the patients in La Charité Hospital in Paris who had been hospitalised for symptoms which although not recognised then, would now be diagnosed as lead poisoning. He showed that all the patients were involved in occupations which exposed them to lead. Some sixty years later Tanquerel des Planches looked at admissions to the same hospital in the years 1830-38. Of the 1213 patients admitted suffering from lead colic, 490 were employed in the manufacture of lead compounds, 390 were painters, 61 were potters, 55 were copper and bronze founders, 35 were lapidaries, 25 were refiners, 14 were plumbers, 11 worked in lead shot factories, and 8 were glaziers or worked in glass factories (quoted by Nriagu, 1983). This indicates that at that time lead poisoning was very predominantly an occupational hazard.

At that time the conditions of employment and the expectations of workers were very different from those held now (Rowe, 1983). Certain jobs carried with them hazards and these were accepted as part of the job. Employment was seen as a financial contract between a worker and his employer and the responsibilities ended there. The state did not intervene. Rowe (1983) quotes a 1747 guide for those contemplating apprenticing their children. On the occupation of making red and white lead the guide states, 'the work is performed by labourers who are sure in a few years to become paralytic by the Mercurial Fumes of the lead; and seldom live more than a dozen Years in the Business.' Charles Dickens summed up the expectations of lead workers in a passage from *The Uncommercial Traveller*:

> Some of them gets lead-pisoned soon, and some of them gets lead-pisoned later, and some but not many, niver; and 'tis all according to the constitooshun, Sur, and some constitooshuns is strong and some is weak.

The conditions in the lead industry were no worse than in many other occupations, and better than some. Unlike the mills and the mines very few children were employed. When the state did start to intervene with legislation and regulations to control the conditions of employment, the lead industry was investigated but little affected. It was not until 1882 after publicity on several deaths of employees in lead works, that questions were asked in Parliament, and a report on white lead factories was prepared. This resulted in the 1883 *Factory and Workshop Act* which laid down special rules for white lead factories. This was followed some time later by a more thorough enquiry into the lead industry by a Home Office committee. The result of this was that from 1896 the minimum age for the employment of women was raised to twenty, and women were prohibited from working in contact with white lead (Rowe, 1983). Oliver (1914) states that these regulations considerably decreased the number of cases of plumbism in females. Nevertheless the figures he quotes for North Staffordshire pottery workers in 1898, two years after the regulations came into force, show that lead poisoning was still a real hazard, with 12 per cent of females, and 5 per cent of male workers being affected. When one considers that Oliver says of white lead workers, 'although they are pale and unhealthy looking, and although on their gums a delicate blue line is observed, these men are not suffering from plumbism. They are all able to follow their employment', it is likely that his criteria for diagnosis of plumbism involved considerable incapacity, and perhaps a degree of paralysis, so the figures for lead poisoning he gives are almost certainly an underestimate by present day criteria.

There were other hazards for lead workers. The rate of spontaneous abortion, stillbirth, and premature delivery was high in female lead workers, and in females whose husbands were lead workers, and infant mortality was high in children of lead workers (Oliver, 1914). Oliver claimed that some women in white lead factories used pregnancy to protect their own health. He says, 'they maintained that child-rearing relieved them of the risks of becoming lead-poisoned, for they passed on the lead to the foetus in utero. The infant died, but the mother's body had parted with the lead'.

Lead poisoning in children unrelated to occupational exposure was fortunately a rare hazard. In 1892 Gibson and colleagues in Australia reported on ten cases of lead colic in children. It took twelve years before lead paint in the children's houses was identified as the source of the poison. Gibson noted, in a paper published in 1904, that this form of lead poisoning was preventable, he noted also the seasonal variation of the plumbism, and that children were at particular risk through the route from house dust and dirt, to hand, to mouth (Lin-Fu, 1980). These observations, like others in the history of lead toxicity, were forgotten for more than half a century.

References

Cordero, H.G. and Tarring, L.H. (1960) *Babylon to Birmingham*, Quin Press, London.

Gilfillan, S.C. (1965) Lead poisoning and the fall of Rome; *J. Occup. Med.*, 7, 53-60.

Krysko, W.W. (1979) *Lead in History and Art*, Verlag, Stuttgart.

Lead Development Association (1974) *Technical Notes on Lead: Production Properties and Uses*. Lead Development Association, London.

Lin-Fu, J.S. (1980) Lead poisoning and undue lead exposure in children: History and current status. In H.L. Needleman (ed.) *Low Level Lead Exposure: the Clinical Implications of Current Research*, Raven Press, New York.

Lucas, A. and Harris, J.R. (1962) *Ancient Egyptian Materials and Industries*, 4th edn, Arnold, London.

McCord, C.P. (1953) Lead and lead poisoning in Early America: Benjamin Franklin

and lead poisoning. *Ind. Med. Surg.*, *22*, 393-9.
— (1954) Lead and lead poisoning in Early America: Clinical lead poisoning in the Colonies. *Ind. Med. Surg.*, *23*, 120-5.
Major, R.H. (1945) *Classic Descriptions of Disease*, 3rd edn, Thomas, Illinois.
Nriagu, J.O. (1983) *Lead and Lead Poisoning in Antiquity*, Wiley, New York.
Oliver, T. (1914) *Lead Poisoning: from the Industrial, Medical and Social Points of View.* Lewis, London.
Pulsifer, W.H. (1888) *Notes for a History of Lead.* Van Nostrand, New York.
Rowe, D.J. (1983) *Lead Manufacturing in Britain.* Croom Helm, London.
Schadewaldt, H. (1967) Verwendung von Bleirohren fur Twinkwasseranlagen? *Munchener Medizinische Wochenschrift*, *109*, 36, 1876-7.
Tylecote, R.F. (1976) *A History of Metallurgy.* The Metals Society, London.
Waldron, H.A. (1973) Lead poisoning in the Ancient World. *Med. Hist.*, *17*, 391-9.

3 THE USES OF LEAD TODAY

Marie Anne Urbanowicz

One of the main reasons for the importance of lead in the world today is that it finds its way, in one form or another, into so many facets of modern life. The automobile industry probably accounts for the largest proportion of lead used, principally in the manufacture of storage batteries and petrol/gasoline additives but also in the solders used for joints and in other ways. Lead is also used for the sheathing of telegraph, telephone and power cables and, although other materials are being increasingly used, cable sheathing remains a major outlet for lead particularly in some European countries. A significant proportion of lead is used in the building industry in the form of sheet and pipes. Lead, in small quantities, in the form of solder and bearings, finds its way into a very wide range of products from car engines to washing machines. It is used in paints, radiation shielding, plastics, ceramics, make-up and in a number of other applications.

The use of lead today runs to over five million metric tons as compared with about four and a half million metric tons in 1975 (Table 3.1). Over the past four or five years, the amount of lead

Table 3.1: Consumption of Refined Lead: World Totals (thousand metric tons). Accounting is based on the consumption of refined pig lead and the lead content of antimonial lead. Remelted pig lead and remelted antimonial lead are excluded

	1975	1978	1980	1982	Jan-Mar 1983
Europe	1411.3	1623.5	1681.8	1571.0	(400)
Africa	73.9	81.6	92.6	97.8	(17.3)
Asia	380.6	506.8	588.5	547.6	(84.4)
America	1433.4	1754.3	1461.7	1432.3	(341.4)
Australasia	81.0	80.6	86.1	72.5	(15.8)
Total Western	3380.2	4046.8	3880.7	3721.2	(910.4)
Other (Eastern block China, Cuba)	1222.80	1423.3	1466.4	1479.2	
World Totals	4603	5470.1	5347.1	5200.4	

Source: World Metal Statistics September 1983

Table 3.2: Refined Lead — Principal Consumers (1982)

Country	Lead (thousand metric tons)	Percentage of World Consumption	
USA	1106.2	21.3	
USSR	810	15.6	
Japan	354	6.8	60
Germany FR	333.2	6.4	
UK	271.9	5.2	
Italy	243	4.7	
China	215	4.0	
France	194.5	3.7	
Bulgaria	120	2.3	
Yugoslavia	115.7	2.2	
Spain	102.7	2.0	
Germany DR	100	1.9	
Total	3966.2	76.2	

Source: World Metal Statistics, 1983

used has fallen slightly and this seems largely due to the fall in consumption in the USA and the UK. Lead is used to some extent by most countries but six countries account for 60 per cent of the world's consumption. If six more countries are added, 76 per cent of the world's consumption of lead is accounted for (Table 3.2).

Before being used in the manufacture of products, lead or lead alloy is treated in a number of ways (Figure 3.1). If lead compounds are required, the lead undergoes the appropriate chemical treatment. For applications such as bearings, some lead sheet, shot and type a casting method is used. Originally this was done by casting molten lead on to a sand bed and although a small amount of lead sheet is still produced in this way, casting is now carried out by more modern methods. An example is the continuous casting method where a rotating water-coated drum is partially immersed in a bath of molten lead and picks up a layer of solid metal. A large proportion of lead sheet is manufactured on rolling mills. Where lead pipes or sheaths are required, these are produced by the extrusion of solid metal at a raised temperature on presses capable of producing long lengths of pipe to very close tolerances. A number of special processes have also been developed for the treatment of lead for particular purposes.

Figure 3.1: Manufacture of Major Lead Products

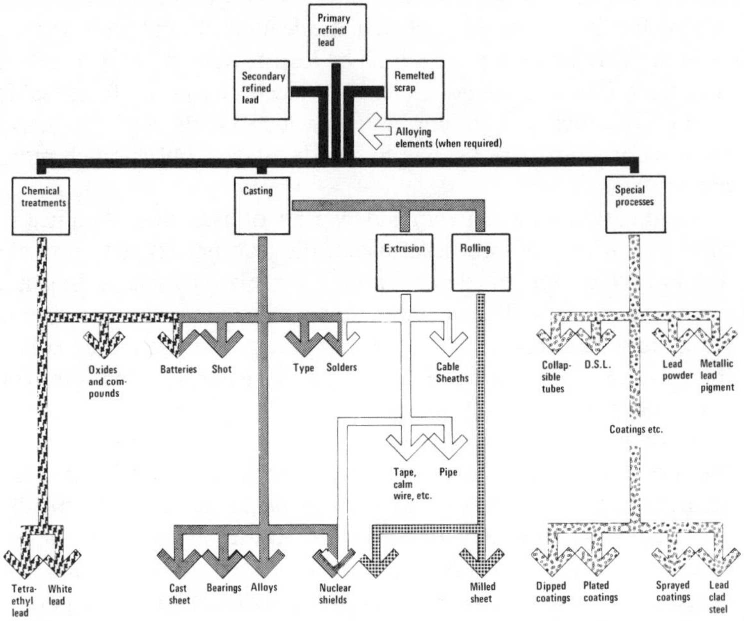

Source: Lead Development Association (1975)

Storage Batteries

Lead-acid batteries are the largest outlet for lead throughout the world (Table 3.3). Both the metallic and compound forms of lead are used in about equal proportions. The lead battery usually comprises a hard rubber or plastic box containing lead-antimony alloy grids into which lead oxide pastes are pressed to form 'plates'. The lead oxides used are generally litharge (PbO), red lead (Pb_3O_4) and grey oxide (PbO_2). The plates are immersed in a solution of sulphuric acid and form an electric cell which produces electricity from the chemical reactions which occur. These reactions are reversible so that the battery can be recharged. Lead is eminently suitable for use in batteries, because of its conductivity and resistance to corrosion. When alloyed with antimony lead is also able to resist the mechanical stresses associated both with the chemical changes within the paste and with the conditions of use of the battery such as the vibration of cars and trucks. The manufacture of the intricate grid required to support and hold the paste is also facilitated by the fact that the lead-antimony alloy is very fluid at fairly low temperatures. The lead battery is likely to retain its position as a convenient source of electricity in the foreseeable future. The nickel-cadmium battery, which excels at giving heavy current for short periods, has some advantages, but is much more expensive.

Lead batteries have a very wide variety of uses other than just in motor vehicles. An important use of the lead battery is to provide a stand-by source of electric power for places such as hospital operating theatres, life-support systems, on-line computer systems, banks and airports. A recent development has been the mobile intensive care unit for babies used when transfer between wards or even hospitals becomes necessary. The lead battery provides a dependable source of electricity in these situations. Another use of the lead battery is to provide power for boats and electric road vehicles (e.g. milk floats). More use is being made of electrically powered boats especially in the leisure industry as they are quieter, cheaper and create minimal pollution problems. About 35 000 low speed electric road vehicles are in use in Britain. They are particularly suitable where small distances are travelled and frequent stops made. Electric vehicles are extensively used at airports, for milk delivery, and for fork-lift trucks. Lead batteries have been developed recently which will allow an electric vehicle a fifty mile range at 50 m.p.h. and the industry hopes to expand the market for electric vehicles. Lead batteries are also used in miners' safety lamps, wheelchairs and invalid carriages and in new developments such as the battery-assisted bicycle.

Table 3.3: Principal Uses of Lead — 1981 (percentage of the total lead consumption for each country)

	Batteries	Tetra-ethyl lead	Chemicals	Cable sheathing	Sheet and pipe
Germany	43		27	8	15
UK	29	21		7	20
France	50	6	14	7	9
Italy	36	4	20	15	13
USA	66	9.5	7	1	2.4
Japan	54		18	10	6

Sources: Lead and Zinc Statistics, 1983; World Metal Statistics, 1983

Lead in Petrol/Gasoline

Lead, in the form of tetra-ethyl lead (TEL) and tetramethyl lead (TML), is added in small quantities to petrol to increase its octane rating and thus to prevent the phenomenon known as 'knocking'. In the petrol engine, the fuel and air are premixed using a carburettor or fuel injector so that the mixture in the combustion chamber is homogeneous. Combustion then takes place progressively across the chamber starting from the spark plugs. The fuel mixture furthest from the spark plugs, known as the end gas, is subject to compression and heating for longer than in any other location and is brought to an abnormal state of partial oxidation. This partially oxidised fuel mixture can then ignite spontaneously at great speed and this is known as 'knocking'. At low engine revolutions this is not too serious, although damage is caused to the piston heads and other engine parts, but at high speeds knocking can be dangerous as it may be inaudible, sudden, and may result in the engine seizing up. The presence or absence of knock for a given design of engine is determined by the combustion quality or 'octane number' of the petrol, the higher the octane number the higher the compression ratio possible without knocking occurring.

Octane quality can be improved by intensive refining of the crude oil but this is more expensive and significantly less petrol is produced from any given amount of crude oil. Sixty years ago, it was found that adding organic lead compounds (lead alkyls) to petrol was a convenient and cheap method of boosting octane quality. The lead compounds delay the partial oxidation of end gas so that the engine can operate at higher compression ratios before knocking occurs. To this day no cost-effective alternatives to lead as an anti-knock additive have been discovered except for methylcyclopentadienyl manganese tri-carbonyl (MMT) which is associated with potential health risks and is banned in the USA at present. The diesel engine, which works on a slightly different principle and uses diesel fuel does not have the problem of knocking. However diesel fuel could meet only part of the total demand for fuel. It is now possible to produce engines which can run efficiently on unleaded petrol and due to the concern over the toxicity of lead expelled in exhaust gases, many countries are moving towards the use of lead-free petrol. In the EEC, there are maximum and minimum levels of lead in petrol of 0.4 g/l and 0.15 g/l.

The minimum is imposed to maintain easy trade and movement between member countries, 0.15 g/l being considered the least lead addition needed to ensure that current motor vehicles can continue to operate. The Royal Commission Report (1983) in the UK recommends that negotiations be commenced within the EEC to remove the minimum restriction and to initiate a move to unleaded petrol. Over the next few years the use of lead in petrol is likely to fall steadily.

Lead in Building

Lead has, for many years, been used in building. Many famous buildings, notably cathedrals, have lead roofs. In the United

Figure 3.2: Lead Roof of New Law Courts, Winchester

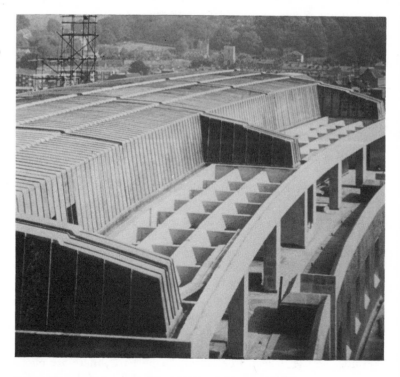

Source: Photograph courtesy of the Lead Development Association

Kingdom in particular there is a tradition of using lead in building and even today it is used in a number of ways. The consumption of lead for sheet and pipes in the United Kingdom is about 54 000 metric tons per year (19 per cent of the total consumption).

Lead Sheet

Lead sheet is useful in building because of its softness and exceptional malleability (see also Chapter 1). It is easy to work at normal temperatures and its strength and durability can be improved by appropriate fixing or by the addition of small amounts of other metals to form alloys. Lead is resistant to corrosion and requires little maintenance. When lead sheet is first exposed to air it forms a surface film of oxide which then reacts with atmospheric carbon dioxide to form a patina of lead carbonate. This patina gradually becomes a strongly adhesive film and is insoluble in normal atmospheric moisture thus preventing penetration of moisture into the metal.

There are now materials available that combine the properties of pure lead with mechanical strength. Two of these are lead-clad steel sheet (steel sheet and lead sheet bonded together), and dispersion strengthened lead (lead sheet in which small amounts of foreign materials have been uniformly dispersed). These materials increase the range of applications of lead.

Lead sheet is used widely for various forms of flashings (Figure 3.3) and weatherings, used to make watertight those parts of buildings that are vulnerable to the ingress of rain. As lead is very malleable, it is ideal for flashings and weatherings that need to fit close to the adjoining structure for effective and lasting watertightness. Lead sheet is used for cladding external walls and recently there has been a resurgence of its traditional use for covering pitched roofs designed as architectural features of buildings. A major advantage of using lead in this way is that it gives a long low-maintenance life to the fabric of buildings. Because of its density and low rigidity, lead is a very effective barrier to the transmission of airborne sound and is often used for this purpose. The lead sheet may be adhesively bonded to plywood or other building board for ease of handling. Lead is also used in various materials for the reduction of noise in industry and from engines.

Lead Pipe

Lead pipes, manufactured by extrusion, were used extensively for

Figure 3.3: Lead Chimney Flashings

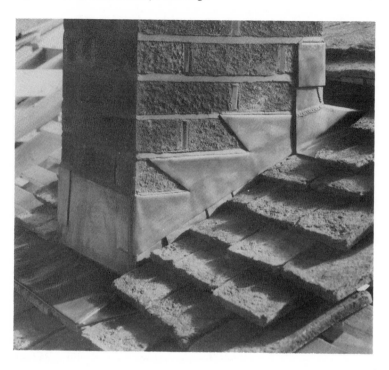

Source: Photography courtesy of the Lead Development Association

all forms of domestic plumbing in the past. However, as cheaper alternatives became available (notably copper and plastic) so, since about 1945 the use of lead pipe has diminished. Currently lead pipes are used only in special applications where corrosion resistance and the ease of manipulation are the important factors. For example, lead is often the most appropriate material for laboratory plumbing. It is also used where short connections need to be made between a rigid pipe and an appliance, for example to wash basins and baths, and to gas meters. Lead continues to be used in solders employed in joining copper pipes in modern plumbing systems.

Cable Sheathing

Lead has been used for the sheathing of telegraph cables since 1845, for telephone cables since 1865 and for power cables since about 1880. Plastic sheathing/insulation is now increasingly replacing lead especially in the USA and Canada. However, the use of lead in cable sheathing continues to be an important outlet for the metal particularly in Europe and some developing countries. In the UK approximately 21 000 tons of lead (7 per cent of total consumption) was used in the manufacture of cable sheathing in 1982.

Lead sheaths are produced by the well-established metalworking process of extrusion. The use of lead provides a durable, impervious sheath, preventing the ingress of moisture. As lead has a low extrusion temperature, it can easily be applied to cables without harming the insulating materials (often paper) which separate the sheath from the conductors at the centre. Cable sheathing is used in a variety of situations and under varied conditions. For example, cables may need to be transported very long distances over difficult terrain, may be laid close to railway bridges, heavy traffic or machinery and may be subject to vibration stresses. The material used must therefore be capable of enduring these varied conditions. The use of various alloys improves lead's performance, the alloy selected varying with the particular use intended. Different alloys have been developed by different countries for cable sheathing. Lead is soft and flexible and can thus withstand the repeated coiling and straightening operations necessary in installation. Little or no maintenance of lead sheathing is required, an important factor in many situations where access is difficult.

Solder and Fusible Alloys

Lead is used in a wide range of products, often in very small quantities, in the form of solder, the main use of which is for joining components together. There are four methods of joining: mechanical (with bolts, rivets, etc.), adhesive bonding, welding and soldering. Welding uses the base metal itself under the influence of heat and/or pressure to form the joint whereas soldering employs another metal, applied in the molten state, to join the two surfaces.

Solders may be applied at various temperatures depending on the metal or alloy used and are classified according to their working temperature. Lead and lead alloys (often lead-tin alloys) are principally used in the solders which have the lowest melting points. Varying the composition of the alloy varies the melting temperature and the properties of the solder. There are two main types of solder as far as melting or freezing modes are concerned. A eutectic soft solder melts completely to a free-flowing liquid at a certain temperature and is therefore used where excessive heat is to be avoided and where a liquid is required to penetrate small gaps (e.g. in electronics). The other type of solder (e.g. 70 per cent lead, 30 per cent tin) goes through a 'pasty' stage over a certain range of temperatures, and is therefore used by plumbers and cable joiners and for car body fillings. Lead-based solders have a wide range of applications. Some of these are in the telecommunications industry, the generation and distribution of electric power, the supply of water and gas, the manufacture of containers for anything from food to petrol and paint, the manufacture of vehicles, radio and television and even down to the smallest electric light bulb.

The use of solder in canning food deserves special mention as this is a direct source of lead for humans. In the USA, the Nutrition Foundation's Expert Advisory Committee concluded that the contribution of canned foods to the lead intake of children is 17 to 28 per cent of dietary lead. Regulations are becoming increasingly more stringent for the amount of lead solder permissible in canning and this use of lead will be phased out over the next few years.

By adding further suitable alloying metals to the lead-tin alloys known as soft solders, fusible alloys which melt at much lower temperatures can be obtained. These fusible alloys are often used in safety devices where the low melting point and softness and weakness of the alloy near its melting temperature are employed to good effect. An example is the use of a fusible alloy in automatic sprinklers where a valve holding back the flow of water is held shut by a mechanical component which is soldered in position with a fusible alloy. In the event of fire, as the temperature rises and approaches the melting point of the alloy, so the soldered component fails and releases the water. Fusible alloys are used in other safety devices such as pressure valves and combined temperature/pressure safety plugs. They are also used as solders where low working temperatures are essential, in the production of brass pressings such as vehicle radiator tanks, assembly jigs and the production of artificial jewellery.

Printing

Lead-tin-antimony alloys are used in the production of printing metals. These alloys are used as they melt completely to form a free-flowing liquid which easily fills all the intricate patterns in the moulds and then, on solidifying, are hard-wearing. The antimony in the alloy also reduces the freezing contraction of the cast type thus giving better accuracy in size. Lead may be used in another way in printing — Hankin *et al.* (1973) found that the coloured inks used in magazine illustrations contain high amounts of lead.

Lead in Bearings

Every moving part in industry, transport or the home employs bearings of some sort. Bearings fall generally into two classes — ball bearings and the associated roller bearings and plain bearings. Lead is often used in plain bearings although in small amounts so that this application of lead accounts for only a small percentage of the total used. However, the number of different applications is very great, and one of the most widespread uses of lead is in bearings, from car engines to rolling mills, flyovers to washing machines.

A bearing is a means by which a load or force is transmitted between two parts which are in motion relative to each other. In a plain bearing the movement is between two surfaces in sliding contact, one of which is normally made of a 'bearing material' chosen for its ability to minimise friction and wear and to avoid seizure or failure by distortion or fatigue. A lubricant is normally used to reduce friction and wear. In most cases, only a relatively thin layer of bearing material is used, mounted on a stronger material as a supporting base. This main structural member is normally steel or bronze. Lead alloys are often used as the bearing material, usually the 'white metal' or 'babbit' bearings containing lead-tin-antimony, alloys of lead and copper and, more recently, aluminium-lead alloys. For special applications where lubrication is either inconvenient or even impossible, special dry bearings are used which have lead dispersed in plastic materials.

Lead in Atomic Energy

Lead is one of the three principal shielding materials used in the field of atomic energy today, the others being concrete and steel. There are four main types of radiation: alpha rays (helium nuclei), beta rays (electrons), gamma rays (electromagnetic radiation) and neutrons (which form part of the nucleus of an atom). The first two types are easily stopped by materials such as perspex, but the second two are highly penetrative forms of radiation and require more complex shielding which is both dense and massive. Where space is not a problem, for example for reactors in power stations, concrete is often used. Where space is more important as in atomic ships and submarines, lead is more likely to be used. It is also commonly used in laboratories and hospitals where radioactive materials are generally handled by remote control from behind a wall of lead bricks. Lead compounds are used in the glass in shielding partitions to permit safe viewing and X-ray machines are normally installed in rooms lined with sheet lead. Lead powder is incorporated into plastic and rubber sheeting to provide a material for protective clothing. Spent reactor fuel is removed for disposal in lead containers and small amounts of radioactive isotope are also transported where necessary in lead containers. In the field of atomic energy lead is normally used in the form of cast or rolled lead sheet, but some extruded lead, shot, wool and glass are also used. New uses are still being developed and the use of lead in safety precautions in this field is likely to expand.

Lead in Paint

Lead pigments have been used in paints from early days and their merits and advantages were known empirically long before any theoretical explanation was possible. Other materials have now been developed and since 1945 much less lead has been used in paints. Modern paint consists mainly of a solvent, binder and pigment. The solvent is water for most emulsion paints used in the home and the binder is a polyeuric resin which forms a thin coherent film when the solvent evaporates. Oil-based paints contain a drier which is normally organic lead or other metal compound and this reduces the drying time from several days to a few hours. Some lead pigments are still used in paints although not usually for emulsion paints designed for internal domestic use. The use of lead in paints in the past often lead to lead poisoning and even today many cases of lead poisoning, especially in children, can be traced back to the ingestion of old flaking paint in pre-war houses and buildings. In the UK, the lead content in paint in industry has been controlled since 1927 although the lead content of paint and related materials available to the general public is not controlled by statute. There is a voluntary agreement between the Government and the Paintmakers' Association to put warning labels on tins of paint containing more than one per cent total lead in the dry film, but there is no control on imported paints. However, a European Community Directive (1977) which concerns the classification, packaging and labelling of paints, primers, varnishes and similar products is due to be implemented shortly.

Red lead (Pb_3O_4) continues to play a major role in rust-inhibiting primary paints applied direct to untreated iron and steel, for example on ships. Paints made from calcium plumbate dry quickly, form tough films with adequate covering power and are unique in their ability to adhere well to zinc and galvanised steel. Metallic lead is increasingly used as a pigment. These paints are generally used in areas such as industrial buildings, shipping and cable protection. Lead chromate, producing a strong yellow colour

Table 3.4: Lead Content of Some Paints on Sale in the UK

Paint	Total lead in dry paint film ($\mu g/g$)
Toy paint	<50
Modern decorative gloss	2 500-3 000
White lead gloss	44 000
White lead undercoat	71 000
White lead primer	448 000
Pink primer	476 000
Red lead paint	661 000

Source: Paintmakers' Association of Great Britain Limited

has been largely replaced by other pigments for most purposes but continues to be used widely in road markings. However, the Royal Commission on Environmental Pollution (1983) recommended that this use of lead should be phased out, and in November 1984 it was reported that the Paintmakers' Association, representing more than 90 per cent of the British industry, has assured the Department of the Environment that lead will be phased out of their products.

Miscellaneous Uses of Lead

In the USA, 5 per cent of the total lead consumption is used in the manufacture of ammunition and it is used to a lesser degree in other countries too. Cast lead is used in lead shot, balance and fishing weights and although no acceptable substitutes for these currently exist, both the Nature Conservancy Council and the Royal Commission recommend phasing out the use of lead and the development of possible alternatives. Lead and its alloys are also used in making yacht keels, canes for leaded windows, wire, imitation jewellery, ornamental castings, seals, collapsible tubes and seatings for manhole covers. Another important use is in certain plastics such as poly vinyl chloride (PVC) where lead compounds (e.g. lead carbonate or lead silicate) are used as stabilisers to extend the range of temperatures over which they can be processed. Lead dithiocarbonate is used as an accelerator in the manufacture of rubber. It is used in glazing for pottery and earthenware, and this may present a hazard especially when the glazing is not carried out properly. Although prohibited in the UK, lead continues to be used in make-up particularly in Oriental countries.

Products, other than those in which lead has been used specifically, may also contain lead either because some of the component parts contain lead or machinery containing lead or lead solder has been used in their manufacture. Thus wine and other beverages and foods often contain appreciable amounts of lead resulting from the production process or solder in containers and caps. Sewage sludge often contains appreciable amounts of lead (via plumbing and waste) and when treated may be used as an agricultural fertiliser. Large quantities of lead can be found in illicitly distilled whisky, particularly in the south eastern parts of the USA, as the condensers used are often discarded car radiators which contain lead in soldered joints. Cigarettes contain some lead, probably due to the use in the past of lead arsenate as an insecticide in tobacco fields.

A large proportion of lead waste is recovered and recycled in secondary lead smelters (Table 3.5). Probably only a very small fraction of the lead used in sheeting, cable, printing and batteries is ever released to the environment except in localised ways (e.g. scrapyards). The combustion of alkyl lead additives in motor fuels is a major source of lead in the environment, the amount varying from country to country with the number of cars in use and the proportion of lead permitted in petrol. It is uncertain how much lead is released from the various lead-containing items which are subjected to weathering or are decomposed over time, although there is evidence which shows that lead from paint significantly affects the content of lead in dust and soil near older houses. The use of lead pipes, PVC pipes, glazed ceramics and cans with lead-antimony solders may all significantly affect domestic water, food and drink. How lead from these sources contributes to environmental pollution and to the uptake of lead in humans is described in detail later in this book.

Table 3.5: Recovery of Lead Products

Product	Life cycle (years)	Product recovery (%)	Recoverable lead (%)
Batteries:			
Automobile	3-4 ⎫		95-97
Traction	5 ⎬	At least 90	
Stationary	20 ⎭		
Sheet	up to 100	80-90 ⎫	
Pipe	50	70-80 ⎬	98-100
Cable sheathing	40	50 ⎭	
Alloys:			
Solder	varies with product ⎫	20-30	
Bearings	in which used ⎬		
Type metal	indefinite — constantly recirculating	5% of annual consumption returned as skimmings and residues from melting operations	98-100

Source: Lead Development Association, London

References

European Community Directive 77/728/EEC (1977) *Official Journal of the European Communities*, L303, 23-32.

Hankin, L., Heichel, G.H. and Botsford, R.A. (1973) Lead poisoning from coloured printing inks. *Clin. Paediatr.*, *12*, 654-5.

Lead and Zinc Study Group (1983) *Lead and Zinc Statistics*, Lead and Zinc Study Group.

Lead Development Association (1975) *Technical Notes on Lead* Lead Development Association, London.

Metal Statistics (1971-81) 69th edn, W. Bauer, (ed.), Metallgesellschaft AG.

Nature Conservancy Council (1981) *Lead Poisoning in Swans* NCC, London.

Royal Commission on Environmental Pollution (1983) *Ninth Report, Lead in the Environment*, HMSO, London.

WHO (1977) *Environmental Health Criteria 3: Lead*, WHO, Geneva.

World Metal Statistics (Sept. 1983) World Bureau of Metal Statistics, London.

4 THE MEASUREMENT OF LEAD

Philippe Grandjean and Richard Lansdown

Lead in the Body

The Body Burden

To speak of a body lead burden is to some extent meaningless because the toxic effects depend on the location of lead within the body. As is discussed further in Chapter 5 lead is stored to different extents in various tissues. For example, lead only stays for a limited period in the blood, and after about one month, only one-half of the original lead is still circulating in the blood. In other words, the half-life of lead in the blood is about thirty days. Several 'soft' organs show a half-life of a few months. In particular, the brain retains lead for a much longer time than does the blood, and this fact may be a partial explanation for the particular susceptibility of the central nervous system. The skeleton stores lead for a much longer time, and in adults the half-life is more than ten years. It is less in children due to the more intensive remodelling of the skeleton in the growing body. Measurement of lead in different tissues must therefore be interpreted in relation to the retention time of the lead in that particular tissue.

Blood Analysis

For assessment of lead in the body, the most widely used method is the measurement of lead in blood. Either capillary or venous blood can be used; the former is easier to obtain but more susceptible to contamination, and the latter is therefore usually preferred. A standardised procedure must be used for the collection, storage, transport and analysis of blood to avoid contamination and other errors, as discussed below in the section on analysis (Aitio, 1981; see also Chapter 14 on methodological issues for a discussion of the further implications). The lead concentration is usually expressed as micrograms per hundred millilitres ($\mu g/100\,ml$ or $\mu g/dl$), where one microgram is a millionth of a gram, and a millilitre is one thousandth of a litre. An expected average blood lead concentration in urban children in the UK would be about 12 or 13 $\mu g/100\,ml$; very few such children would have concentrations

41

Figure 4.1: Haem Biosynthetic Pathway. The two enzymatic steps most sensitive to inhibition by lead are indicated by asterisks. The results are measurable enzyme inhibition, excess excretion of aminolaevulinic acid in the urine and accumulation of abnormal haemoglobin with zinc protoporphyrin in the red blood cells

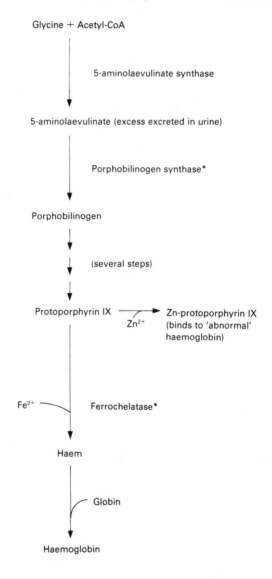

higher than 35 µg/100ml. (See also Chapter 6 on the distribution of lead.) Recently several countries have adopted a new unit system, namely the SI units. According to this agreement, concentrations should be expressed on a molar basis. Thus, blood lead levels are reported as micromoles per litre (µmol/l). A typical blood lead level of, say, 10 µg/100ml would then be expressed as 0.5 µmol/l, the conversion factor being 20.7. In some reports, the blood lead concentration has been expressed in relation to volume of red blood cells, because almost all the lead in blood is associated with the cells. The lead concentration in whole blood is then divided by the haematocrit which usually is about 0.40-0.45 (see also Appendix).

The lead level in blood may also be assessed by indirect methods, because lead interferes with the production of haemoglobin, the oxygen-carrying pigment of the blood. This biochemical effect is partly due to inhibition of the enzyme aminolaevulinic acid dehydratase, abbreviated ALAD (although a more correct name is porphobilinogen synthase). This inhibition may be detected at blood lead levels of 5-10 µg/100ml and the enzyme activity decreases in an exponential fashion when the blood lead level increases (Berlin and Schaller, 1974). The biochemical interference also results in the formation of unfinished haemoglobin molecules which contain zinc protoporphyrin instead of haem (Lamola and Yamane, 1974). The most frequent abbreviations are ZPP (zinc protoporphyrin) and EPP (erythrocyte protoporphyrin). This analysis is much simpler than direct analysis of the lead concentration, and the test result is not affected by possible contamination with lead during the sampling. Each red blood cell contains an amount of ZPP which is a testimony of the lead level when the cell developed, and a blood sample normally contains cells which are between 1 and 120 days old. Thus the ZPP level indicates the average lead level during the last four months. However, a significant increase in protoporphyrin may not be detected in children until the average lead concentration in the blood has exceeded 15, or perhaps 20, µg/100ml (Piomelli *et al.*, 1982). Also, some children may be more susceptible to this interference than are others, and iron deficiency by itself may cause a considerable increase in protoporphyrin. Therefore, even though the ZPP or EPP is essentially a measure of a chronic metabolic effect of lead, the use of this method for screening purposes at lead levels averaging about 15 µg/100ml is not recommended (Royal Commission on Environmental Pollution, 1983). At higher levels, and as a supplementary diagnostic test, this method has unique advantages. ALAD rarely adds much additional information to a blood lead measurement. The activity of ALAD is usually expressed in European units according to a European recommendation for the standard conditions of analysis (Berlin and Schaller, 1974). The protoporphyrin concentration is expressed as the content per unit volume of red blood cells or per mole of haemoglobin ($\mu g/100 \, ml$ or $\mu mol/mol$), because protoporphyrin is bound to haemoglobin in the red cells. When the concentration of protoporphyrin is expressed as a molar fraction, it appears that almost one per cent of the haemoglobin under conditions of lead poisoning is bound to zinc protoporphyrin and inactivated.

Urine Analysis

The lead excretion in urine has sometimes been used as an indicator of lead intake. However, proper information must be based on 24-hour urine samples which are frequently difficult to obtain. This problem also relates to other urine analyses, such as the assessment of delta-aminolaevulinic acid (or 5-aminolaevulinic acid) which at high exposure levels is excreted in the urine due to the considerable inhibition of ALAD (Haeger-Aronson, 1971).

Lead in Teeth

Lead analysis of teeth has been recommended as a better measure of long-term lead retention in the body. Details of the storage of lead in teeth are given in Chapter 5, and a further discussion of the methodological points is given in Chapter 14. Although a few researchers have analysed extracted teeth, shed deciduous teeth from 6 to 7-year-old children have been most commonly employed. The unit of measurement usually is micrograms per gram ($\mu g/g$) or parts per million (ppm). Studies in the UK (Smith *et al.*, 1983) and the Federal Republic of Germany (Ewers *et al.*, 1982) have suggested that the mean lead concentration in shed incisors is about 5 $\mu g/g$ with about 90 per cent being below 9 $\mu g/g$. Levels in Denmark appear to be about half as high. Other researchers have preferred to analyse the 'circumpulpal' dentine in the middle of the tooth where higher lead concentrations are retained (Needleman *et al.*, 1979; Grandjean *et al.*, 1984). Such dentine levels in groups of American children have averaged about 50 $\mu g/g$ while a lower average (about 10 $\mu g/g$) has been found in Denmark.

The use of teeth has some practical drawbacks. The investigator obviously has to wait until the child sheds a tooth at 6-7 years of age, or about 6 years later. This disadvantage has been overcome by an X-ray fluorescence method which measures the lead content of the tooth *in situ* but obviously exposes the child to a small dose of radiation (a negligible quantity) (Bloch *et al.*, 1976). Some studies have shown an additional disadvantage in the variation in lead levels from tooth to tooth within the same mouth, and more than one tooth may have to be analysed to obtain an accurate evaluation of the lead retention in a each child (Delves *et al.*, 1982; Grandjean *et al.*, 1984).

The lead concentrations in blood and teeth from the same children are not expected to show any close correlation. The lead in the blood may vary over short periods of time, while the lead in the tooth probably reflects a long-term retention. In addition, both methods are subject to possible errors and bias. Not surprisingly, low correlations of 0.4-0.5 have been reported (Ewers *et al.*, 1982; Smith *et al.*, 1982).

Lead in Hair

The use of hair to measure lead has immediate attraction: it involves no invasive procedures, can be used at any age, and transportation and storage represents no problem. However, the limitations are considerable and have discouraged more widespread use: it is difficult to disentangle what is *in* the hair from what is *on* it (Grandjean, 1984). The unit of measurement is usually µg/g or ppm. Most studies have suggested average lead concentration of a few ppm as a normal background average, but a median of more than 50 ppm has been reported for children living near lead smelters. However, many reports are difficult to evaluate, because contamination from external sources cannot be ruled out and because documented influence by hair colour and hair pigments has not been taken into account. Hair analysis is uniquely useful to investigate relative changes in lead exposure during the past months, in cases where external contamination has been minimal. A hair grows at a rate of about 1 cm per month, and long hair strands have therefore in a few situations been used as calendars of lead intake (Grandjean, 1984).

Environmental Lead

Lead in Air

Lead in air is measured by collecting particulate material on a filter over a period of time and analysing it for the lead content. The volume of air passed through the filter is measured on a pump. The unit of measurement is micrograms of lead per cubic metre ($\mu g/m^3$). Long-term concentrations in rural areas in the UK are usually below 0.15 $\mu g/m^3$, and in most large cities they are below 1.0 $\mu g/m^3$ (Royal Commission on Environmental Pollution, 1983). However, these levels may be exceeded near point sources or close to motorways. For example, a mean level of 9.7 $\mu g/m^3$ was found in the summer of 1979 in the central reservation of the M4 motorway (Colwill and Hickman, 1981), and other studies have found high levels in tunnels and underground parking garages. Inside buildings, lead levels average about 75 per cent of the concentrations outside, higher of course in the summer than in winter. Under the terms of a recent European Economic Community Directive (82/844/EEC), member countries must ensure that lead in air does not exceed an annual average of 2 $\mu g/m^3$ by the end of 1987. A tougher standard applies in the USA: 1.5 $\mu g/m^3$ as a three-month average.

Lead in Dust

The lead content of dust is of particular significance for children who may ingest the lead by sucking dirty fingers, toys or other objects. The unit of measurement is usually $\mu g/g$ or ppm. The concentration in household dust is usually below 1000 $\mu g/g$, but higher levels have been found in the homes of smelter and accumulator factory workers and near motorways. In children of lead workers, increased lead levels in the blood have frequently been associated with lead contents in house dust above 1000 $\mu g/g$ (Baker *et al.*, 1977). In school playgrounds, some local authorities in the UK have found levels of up to 1000 $\mu g/g$, but the highest concentrations, over 12 000 $\mu g/g$, have been documented in car parks and garage forecourts (Harrison, 1979). In 1981 the Greater London Council set a safety limit of 5000 $\mu g/g$ for lead in schools.

Lead in Water

Lead contents of water samples may be determined by direct analysis or by lead detection following preconcentration. Usually the concentration is expressed in micrograms per litre (μg/l) or ppb in American literature (parts per 'billion'). A survey carried out in the UK between 1975 and 1976 by the Department of the Environment showed that most households had lead concentrations of less than 10 μg/l in the daytime samples of tap water. However, the range was up to 300 μg/l and above, with 16 per cent of households between 100 and 300 μg/l, in the Glasgow area where soft water and lead pipes prevail. Also, higher levels may be found in 'first draw' water in the morning. The limit prescribed by a European Economic Community Directive (75/440/EEC) is 50 μg/l.

Analytical Methods

An analytical method encompasses the whole procedure from sampling through storage and transport to sample preparation and detection of the element or compound in question (Aitio, 1981). With trace analysis of lead, the main problem in the initial steps of the analysis is to avoid contamination by lead which is universally present in the everyday environment. Usually a relatively large sample of water, dust, blood, urine or other medium is gathered, and only a small subsample is used for the lead determination with sensitive instrumentation. Between the time of sampling and time of detection of lead, the sample has to be stored, and during the storage time lead may leach out of the sample or traces of lead from the container or stopper may contaminate the sample. This aspect is of particular importance for fluid samples. Containers must be certified to be without significant lead content, such as certain evacuated blood containers which are commercially available. At room temperature, some of the lead from an aqueous solution will become adsorbed onto the walls of the container, but this process is much slower at a low pH and low temperature. Also, some adsorption may occur in frozen blood samples, unless they are kept at a temperature of $-80°$C and preferably in special, pretreated tubes which are less likely to adsorb lead on the walls.

The analysis of samples with very low lead content is only possible when using 'clean laboratory techniques': the laboratory should be constructed with lead-free materials and supplied with filtered air, all personnel should wear special lead-free ('surgical') protective clothing, and all equipment and chemicals should be

Figure 4.2: Equipment for Detection of Lead by Atomic Absorption
Spectrometry

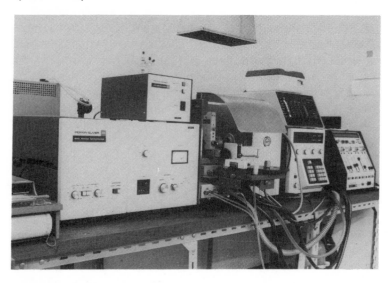

lead-free or cleaned/distilled/purified to prevent lead contamination. Such laboratories are in operation in only a few places in the
world. Some have developed the sophisticated methodology for
the purpose of analysing lead isotopes in lunar rocks, and this
development has now become useful for analysis of lead in sea
water, glacier ice, etc. A laboratory equipped for lead analysis of
biological samples is shown in Figure 4.2.

The preparation of the sample is of particular importance,
because difficulties in the detection method may be avoided by
certain steps in the preparation technique. However, such steps
may also introduce additional contamination. In biological samples
such as blood and urine, the total lead content is of importance,
and a complete digestion of the sample should be achieved,
preferably by wet ashing at a low temperature, because ashing at
high temperatures may cause losses of lead from the sample. In
samples of soil, the total lead content may be of less interest,
because much lead will be insoluble and unavailable for gastrointestinal absorption if ingested. In such cases, the preparation step
would then comprise some sort of extraction procedure, where
'soluble' lead is extracted by a chelating agent or an acid in order
to mimic the processes which occur in the gastrointestinal tract.

Some biological samples, such as teeth, are not homogeneous, and the preparation procedure is of particular importance due to the differential distribution of lead in the dental tissues. The outermost layer of enamel is usually high in lead, and high levels also accumulate in the circumpulpal dentine. Thus, the lead content in a homogenised whole tooth or crown of a tooth is lower than the lead concentration in a sample of circumpulpal dentine or enamel.

Lead is usually detected by means of atomic absorption spectrometry or anodic stripping voltammetry. Two different versions of atomic absorption are usually employed. In the original form, a solution containing lead is injected as an aerosol into a flame in which the lead becomes atomised. The lead atoms then absorb some of the light from a lamp with a lead cathode depending on the amount of lead present in the flame. This absorption at a characteristic wave length is registered by a photocell. A lower detection limit can be obtained by the so-called flameless procedure using an electrothermally heated graphite tube or platform. A small volume of the solution, or even a solid sample, such as a piece of a hair, is placed in the graphite tube or on the platform. Predetermined temperatures for drying, ashing and atomisation are achieved by passing an electric current through the graphite.

In the anodic stripping technique, the positively charged lead ions from the solution are 'plated' on a negatively charged mercury droplet (cathode) over a certain time period. The current is then reversed, and at the characteristic electrochemical potential, lead is then released from the mercury electrode, and the time necessary to release all the lead ions is proportional to the amount of lead originally present in the solution.

These two methods are both useful in the detection of nanogram amounts of lead (Grandjean and Olsen, 1984).

The ALAD enzyme activity is assessed by a biochemical method which measures the amount of porphobilinogen produced under standard conditions (Berlin and Schaller, 1974). The content of delta-aminolaevulinic acid in the urine is usually measured by means of the characteristic light absorption of the complex with Ehrlich's reagent (Haeger-Aronson, 1971). The erythrocyte zinc protoporphyrin is fortunately fluorescent, and the amount in a drop of capillary blood may be determined by front-face fluorimetry (on a 'haematofluorimeter') in a matter of seconds or by conventional spectrofluorimetry after extraction of a blood sample (Grandjean and Lintrup, 1978).

Analytical Validity

Variation of laboratory results originates from changes which take place during sampling, transportation, storage and preparation and from the analytical variation proper (Aitio, 1981). The variation may be divided into two major areas, random variation (lack of precision) and bias (lack of accuracy). The precision is the agreement between duplicate measurements, i.e. repeated analysis of the same sample reveals a uniform result. However, the true value may be different, and accuracy indicates the agreement between the true value and the analytical result. Thus, a very precise analysis may be biased and show a lack of accuracy. On the other hand, an analysis which, on the average, shows a good accuracy, may not necessarily be very precise, because replicate analyses may show large variations. Precision is usually assessed by means of estimates of within-day or day-to-day variation of a (standard) sample. Accuracy is more difficult to estimate, because the true lead content of a sample is rarely known. The recovery of added lead is often a good guide, and the method of standard additions is frequently used: the specimen is analysed in replicate, with a known amount of lead added to one of the subsamples. Recovery may be decreased at atomic absorption analysis, if other substances in the sample cause interference, e.g. due to a matrix effect. Such interference may be adjusted for by means of the standard addition method.

The analyses are usually performed by comparing the signal generated by the sample to the one elicited by a standard. The quality of the standard is therefore of crucial importance. With regard to lead, standards with low concentrations are stable only for short time periods, even when the pH has been adjusted by addition of nitric acid. The standards used for calibration are usually so-called secondary standard solutions of lead in an aqueous solution. Primary standard materials may be biological samples (e.g. freeze dried, homogenised bovine liver) with a certified lead content. A primary standard material for blood lead analysis is not easily available with the low concentrations of lead usually encountered, although reference samples have been circulated by some experienced laboratories.

In order to produce analytical results of high quality, an internal quality control programme in the laboratory should be established. As an initial step, all sources of error should be identified and assessed from collection through transportation, storage, registration, preparation to final detection of lead and calculation and reporting of the result. When the analytical method has become established, and necessary adjustments have been introduced, the accuracy of the method should be assessed by comparison with a reference method, if available, or the previously used method. Interlaboratory comparison studies may also be useful at this stage. The reproducibility of the method under routine conditions should be defined, and the limits of acceptable variation should be set. The means and standard deviations for control materials should be recorded during routine operation. If the limits for acceptable variations are exceeded, the analytical series for that day or that particular run should be discarded, and any errors should be corrected so that optimum conditions may be achieved again. All analyses should be performed in duplicate, and the two duplicates should preferably be interspersed with other samples, standards and control samples. A control sample is a material which is analysed every day as part of the routine procedure. In case of blood lead determination, the control sample may be a large portion of blood obtained from a single individual, separated into a large number of subsamples which are individually frozen. After a number of analyses of this material, experience will indicate the expected mean and standard deviation under routine circumstances. The frequent analysis of this material will therefore be useful to detect if any abnormal performance occurs. In the routine internal quality assurance, detailed recordkeeping is of course of paramount importance.

External quality assessment is a procedure, where a standard material with a known (preferably 'true') lead concentration is distributed to a number of laboratories, and the results are used as an indication of the individual laboratory performance. Acceptable results at such external quality assessment studies are frequently used as a prerequisite for the certification of a laboratory for performing lead analyses. Some studies have, in the past, shown very large variations between a number of laboratories which perform blood lead determinations. More recent experience has shown that interlaboratory variability tends to decrease after repeated participation in such studies. Difficulties have occurred in a few cases when 'spiked' blood portions have been used, perhaps because the added lead was not distributed homogeneously or because some of the lead added was adsorbed onto the walls of the containers. Internal quality control has repeatedly been shown to be a necessary prerequisite for obtaining acceptable results, but poor performance in external quality assessment studies may even occur in cases where the internal quality control programme allegedly is sufficient.

Interpretation

As part of the preventive efforts against undue lead exposure, responsible authorities often rely on acceptable limits or standards. Although such limits may be useful for administrators to separate good from evil, the interpretation of analytical results is a somewhat more complicated matter than mere comparison with an official limit which may have resulted from a compromise decision (Piomelli *et al.*, 1982).

First of all, in the case of biological samples, one needs to assess the relationship to the metabolic model. Which body compartment is represented by the sample analysed? For environmental samples, the following question should be asked: Is the sample representative of the medium from which it was obtained?

Further, the time relationship needs to be evaluated. Lead participates in dynamic processes and is transferred from one part of the body to another, and it may travel between different media of the biosphere. Thus, the question should also be asked: Is the sample representative when seen in a time perspective?

Then analytical validity should be considered. For the individual sample, information should be available on the fate of the sample from collection to the reporting of the analytical result. In particular, contamination is of major interest, because lead is present everywhere and may add to the lead content in the sample, unless stringent precautions have been taken. In addition, the analytical experience and capability of the laboratory should be evaluated, preferably on the basis of its certification or performance in recent external quality control programmes.

Under most circumstances such detailed interpretation is not undertaken and may only rarely be necessary in detail. However, reliance on single analytical values of unknown or dubious origin should certainly be avoided, and the use of analytical results should always be supported by a reference to assessments of the above criteria for prudent interpretation of the results.

References

Aitio, A. (1981) *Quality Control in the Occupational Toxicology Laboratory,* Interim Document 4, World Health Organization, Regional Office for Europe, Copenhagen.

Baker, E.L., Jr., Folland, D.S. Taylor, T.A., Frank, M., Peterson, W., Lovejoy, G., Cox, D., Housworth, J. and Landrigan, P.J. (1977) Lead poisoning in children of lead workers. *N. Engl. J. Med., 296,* 260-1.

Berlin, A. and Schaller, K.H. (1974) European standardized method for the determination of γ-aminolevulinic acid dehydratase in blood. *Zeitschrift für klinische Chemie und klinische Biochemie, 12,* 389-90.

Bloch, P., Garavaglia, G., Mitchell, G. and Shapiro, I.M. (1976) Measurement of lead content of children's teeth *in situ* by X-ray fluorescence. *Phys. Med. Biol., 20,* 56-63.

Colwill, D.M. and Hickman, A.J. (1981) Measurement of particulate lead on the M4 motorway at Harlington, Middlesex. *Transport and Road Research Laboratory Report No. 972.*

Delves, H.T., Clayton, B.E., Carmichael, A., Bubear M. and Smith, M. (1982) An appraisal of the analytical significance of tooth lead measurements as possible indices of environmental exposure of children to lead. *Ann. Clin. Biochem., 19,* 329-37.

Ewers, U., Brockhaus, A., Winneke, G., Freier, I., Jermann, E. and Kraemer, U. (1982) Lead in deciduous teeth of children living in a non-ferrous smelter area and a rural area of the F.R.G. *Int. Arch. Occup. Environ. Health, 50,* 139-51.

Grandjean, P. (1984) Lead poisoning: Hair analysis shows the calendar of events. *Human Toxicol., 3,* 223-8.

Grandjean, P., Hansen, O.N. and Lyngbye, K. (1984) Analysis of lead in circumpulpal dentine of deciduous teeth. *Ann, Clin. Lab. Sci., 14,* 270-5.

Grandjean, P. and Lintrup, J. (1978) Erythrocyte-Zn-protoporphyrin as an indicator of lead exposure. *Scand. J. Clin. Invest., 38,* 669-75.

Grandjean, P. and Olsen, N.B. (1984) Lead in A. Vercruysse (ed.). *Hazardous Metals in Human Toxicology,* Elsevier, Amsterdam, pp. 153-69.

Haeger-Aronson, B. (1971) An assessment of the laboratory tests used to monitor the exposure of lead workers. *Br. J. Indust. Med., 28,* 52-8.

Harrison, R.M. (1979) Toxic metals in street and household dusts. *Sci. Total Environ., 11,* 89-97.

Lamola, A.A. and Yamane, T. (1974) Zinc protoporphyrin in the erythrocytes of patients with lead intoxication and iron deficiency anemia. *Science, 186,* 936-8.

Needleman, H.L., Gunnoe, C.E. Leviton, A., Reed, R., Peresie, H., Maher, C. and Barrett, P. (1979) Deficits in psychologic and classroom performance of children with elevated lead levels. *N. Engl. J. Med., 300,* 689-95.

Piomelli, S., Seaman, C., Zullow, D., Curran, A. and Davidson, B. (1982) Threshold for lead damage to heme synthesis in urban children. *Proc. Nat. Acad. Sci. USA, 79,* 3335-9.

Royal Commission on Environmental Pollution (1983) *Lead in the Environment.* Ninth Report London: HMSO.

Smith, M., Delves, T., Lansdown, R., Clayton, B.E. and Graham, P. (1983) The effects of lead exposure on urban children. Institute of Child Health/University of Southampton study. *Dev. Med. Child Neurol., Suppl. 25,* (5), No. 47.

5   LEAD IN HUMANS

Michael R. Moore

Introduction

The complexity of the relationship between sources of lead exposure and human exposure to lead, is exemplified by the complexity of the homocentric diagrams such as those in the chapter on sources (page 179), or that published by the National Academy of Sciences in the USA (NAS, 1980). Although there has been a dramatic decrease in the number of deaths from lead poisoning through this century which was paralleled by the decrease in the number of notifications of industrial lead poisoning (Waldron and Stofen, 1974), evidence shows that until the late 1960s the quantity of lead that man was being exposed to in his environment was rising (NAS, 1980). This was consistent with the continuing increase in the quantities of alkyl lead used as anti-knock agent in automotive fuels. Since that time, mean blood lead concentrations in the populations of the USA and Germany have been falling (Mahaffey *et al.*, 1979; Sinn, 1981; Annest *et al.*, 1983; Centre for Disease Control, 1982). This has been linked by some authorities with falling sales of leaded petrol. Indeed highly significant regressions have been found between lead in blood and leaded petrol sales (Rabinowitz and Needleman, 1982; 1983; Annest *et al.*, 1983).

When man is exposed to lead he may absorb it by two principal routes. The first of these is by gastrointestinal absorption and this represents the major entry point for lead to the body. The average uptake by this route has been calculated as being around 10-20 per cent (DHSS, 1980). Thus most ingested lead is not in fact absorbed but passes out unchanged in the faeces. There is secondarily, pulmonary absorption. Although a lesser route this has a greater percentage uptake of around 40 per cent. Where lead is absorbed by pulmonary or gastrointestinal absorption it is transported first by blood to soft tissues, in which the half-life is fairly short, i.e. months rather than years, and subsequently to the long half-life, high volume reservoir of bone. Greater than 90 per cent of the total body lead is found in bone as relatively insoluble lead

Figure 5.1: Uptake and Distribution of Lead in a Female Human. The seat of lead deposition in the body is the long bones. Other soft tissues contain much less lead although concentrations in the kidney may be higher as the primary excretory organ of absorbed materials

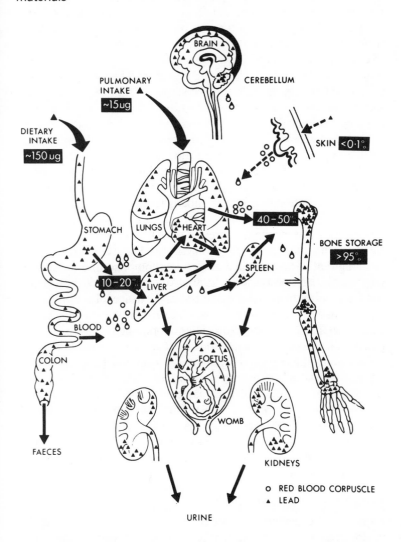

phosphates and in this form the lead does not present a major biohazard (Figure 5.1).

Absorption of Lead from Diet

Although lead is ubiquitously available in the environment, it must be absorbed to become toxic. A number of factors combine to make our ability to predict quantities and rates of absorption and retention extremely inaccurate. This is, however, an area of considerable interest and it is for that reason that there is available a surfeit of information of the effects in laboratory rodents. Because of differences in physiology the quantitative relationship of absorption in rodents certainly cannot be extrapolated to man. There is a 10-fold difference in the rate of absorption from the gut between the laboratory rat and man. Rats absorb around 1 per cent of ingested lead whereas man has been shown to absorb in excess of 10 per cent (Rabinowitz *et al.*, 1976; Blake, 1976; Moore *et al.*, 1979), although it is of interest that rats fed on human diets showed absorption rates of between 3 and 8 per cent, much closer to the normal human figure (Kostial and Kello, 1979). In rats and mice the absorption of lead was initially reported as being independent of dose (Conrad and Barton, 1978) but subsequent investigation has shown that greater dose levels are associated with smaller percentage retention. These results are interpreted as meaning that gastrointestinal absorption comprises more than one process (Keller and Doherty, 1980; Aungst *et al.*, 1981) which is consistent with the processes of intra- and extracellular transport at the intestinal membrane (Blair *et al.*, 1979; Hillburn *et al.*, 1980). There is firstly a carrier-mediated component and secondly, passive diffusion, the major contribution in these circumstances being due to the carrier component (Aungst and Fung, 1981a,b). Ultrastructural autoradiography using lead-210 as tracer showed considerable quantities of lead associated with intestinal cellular organelles (Parmley *et al.*, 1979). Different parts of the gastrointestinal tract will obviously have different levels of lead absorption and studies *in vitro* have shown that jejunal absorption is much greater than that of the duodenum or colon from rats (Gerber and Deroo, 1975).

Factors Influencing Absorption

As might be expected the solubility of lead is a major determinant of absorption. For example large particle size lead metal is less easily absorbed by the gut than small particles (less than 6 μm) (Barltrop and Meek, 1979). A number of other factors contribute to the changes in absorption. Feeding decreases absorption (Garber and Wei, 1974; Aungst and Fung, 1981b; Heard and Chamberlain, 1982) and following food restriction it has been noted that the retention of lead is increased although there was not always an increase in the lead content of the animal (Quarterman *et al.*, 1976). This was examined further by Aungst and Fund (1981) who found that treatment with drugs which alter gastric function influence lead absorption. Propantheline which reduces gastric motility decreased lead absorption and the possibility clearly exists of adaption of absorptive and excretory processes (Kelliher *et al.*, 1973; Morrison *et al.*, 1974; Moore *et al.*, 1975). Animals given a purified diet showed increased susceptibility to lead toxicity because of increased absorption from such diets (Mylroie *et al.*, 1978; Shah *et al.*, 1980; Anders *et al.*, 1982).

Age is also an important determinant of the rate of absorption from the gut. Young animals and human infants all show increased absorption and retention of lead (Kostial *et al.*, 1974; Alexander *et al.*, 1974; Quarterman and Morrison, 1978; Ziegler *et al.*, 1978; Mykkanen and Wasserman, 1981).

Water

Where the concentration of lead in water is high, the actual accumulation of lead by foods from cooking water during the culinary process will increase the total quantity ingested in a more than additive manner (Berlin *et al.*, 1977; Moore *et al.*, 1979; Smart *et al.*, 1981). From Duplicate Diet Study results, the model of the relationship which gave the most satisfactory fit to the observed results for adults was

$$PbB = 18.9 \text{ (weeks intake of lead mg)}^{-3} - 1.4$$

where PbB is the blood lead concentration in mg/100 ml. The important feature of this study was that it indicated that when water lead concentrations were around 100 µg/1 approximately equal quantities of lead would be contributed to the total week's intake from water and from diet and above this figure the principal contribution would be from water (Figure 5.2).

Minerals

Calcium. Of the dietary components most likely to influence lead absorption minerals have been most extensively examined.

Figure 5.2: Blood-Water Lead Relationships in Infancy. These graphs of results from duplicate diet studies in bottle-fed infants show that a curvlinear relationship is the most appropriate. Like adults this can be expressed as a cube-root relationship

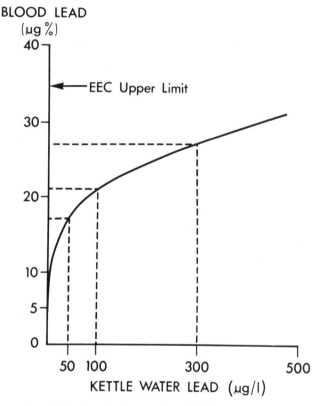

The retention of lead varies inversely with dietary calcium content, and points to two mechanisms acting in the transport of lead from the lumen of the gastrointestinal tract across the gut wall, only one of which is influenced by calcium (Meredith *et al.*, 1977b) (Figure 5.3). In consequence there may well be a basis in mineral deficiency for the development of lead pica in infants (Snowdon, 1977). However, systemic calcium concentrations do not appear to influence lead retention (Quarterman and Morrison, 1975; Meredith *et al.*, 1977b). It has been postulated that calcium and lead share binding sites and absorptive proteins to cause this effect (Barton *et al.*, 1978b) and indeed that iron will act similarly

Figure 5.3: The Influence of Increasing Concentrations of Calcium on the Retention of [203]Lead Chloride in the Rat

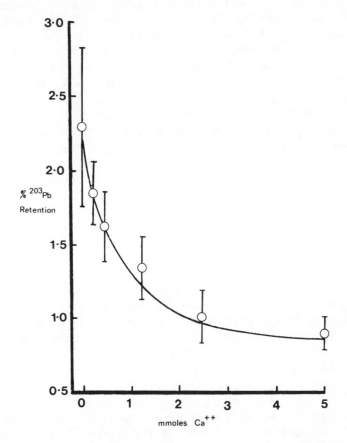

(Barton *et al.*, 1978a). In support of this it has been found that lead inhibits the transport of calcium across the duodenal walls of rats *in vitro* (Gruden *et al.*, 1974) and that lead will interfere further with calcium metabolism, through increases in serum calcium without equivalent rises in calcitonin levels (Peng *et al.*, 1979).

The mechanism for this effect of dietary calcium is little understood. Suggested sites of interaction include competition for absorption in the gastrointestinal tract, increases in excretion by the kidney or competition for storage sites in bone and the influence of vitamin D (Goyer, 1978). Studies using inverted intestinal sack preparations suggest that lead transport into the serosal compartment is related to water movement. Ionic lead utilises the extracellular route to traverse the intestinal barrier. Any process that alters the 'tight' junction between cells will increase lead absorption. Indeed depleted concentrations of calcium and increased acidity which affect this junction have been linked with increased absorption of lead (Blair *et al.*, 1979; Coleman *et al.*, 1978). Lead also interacts with tissue phosphate which removes the lead from the available transport pool. Although dietary phosphate deficiency may significantly increase the lead burden by decreasing intraluminal lead precipitation and increasing its retention by marrow and bone, increased dietary phosphate acts primarily to limit lead absorption (Barton and Conrad, 1981). Since phytate (inositol-hexaphosphate) is the major store of phosphate in plants and since calcium phytate has a great affinity for lead, the combination of these two factors, calcium and phosphorus, means that calcium phytate from plant sources in food provides a natural protective factor against lead toxicity by diminishing absorption (Wise, 1981).

Most other minerals, such as iron (Six and Goyer, 1972), zinc (Conrad and Barton, 1978; Cerklewski and Forbes, 1976; El-Gazzar *et al.*, 1978), copper (Klauder and Petering, 1975), magnesium (Fine *et al.*, 1976; Cerklewski, 1983), diminish lead absorption from the gut. In work on humans low mineral content in the diet increased human uptake of lead by 63.3 per cent. The combination of calcium and phosphorus reduced absorption to 10 per cent (Heard and Chamberlain, 1982).

Vitamin D.   Associated with the absorption of calcium, vitamin D administration also influences lead uptake. Where higher vitamin D concentrations are found, there is enhancement of lead absorption (Smith *et al.*, 1978). However, in lead-poisoned children, vitamin D deficiency is associated with high blood levels (Sorell *et al.*, 1977; Rosen *et al.*, 1980; Box *et al.*, 1981). On the basis of the negative correlation between blood levels and serum levels of 1,25-dihydroxy vitamin D, Rosen *et al.* (1980) concluded that lead impaired the production of this compound or enhanced its conversion into inactive product. In animal studies, cholecalciferol supplementation resulted in a net increase in intestinal absorption of lead (Hart and Smith, 1981) with concurrent changes in the distribution of lead within tissue (Barton *et al.*,

1980). It was also found that such deficiency diminished lead excretion and that single doses of vitamin D accelerated removal of lead from the body even where the element was deposited largely in bone.

The confusion here in many ways typifies the difficulties experienced in examining any one dietary component in isolation. The increase in absorption of lead where vitamin D levels are low almost certainly comes about because of a poor nutritional state of which the low vitamin level is purely an index whereas the increased lead uptake in repletion represents the genuine effect of vitamin D.

Iron. The role of iron in lead absorption is interesting. Animal studies clearly show that in iron deficiency compensatory increases in oral iron absorption is accompanied by an increase in oral lead absorption (Ragan, 1977; Hamilton, 1978; Barton *et al.*, 1978a; Flanagan *et al.*, 1979). For this reason it is perhaps not surprising that supplementation of a lead-containing diet with iron will diminish both the absorption of lead and its toxic effects, although such treatment is ineffective in reversing established lead toxicity (Suzuki and Yoshida, 1979). However, iron absorption is apparently not influenced by increased lead concentrations which would suggest that unlike calcium absorption there is no direct relationship between the transfer of lead and iron across the small intestine of the adult rat (Dobbins *et al.*, 1978; Robertson and Worwood, 1978). The fact remains, however, that iron deficiency does increase the absorption of lead and that iron loading decreases absorption of lead and treatments such as hypertransfusion, endotoxin administration and intravenous injection of iron, which are known to decrease iron absorption, similarly decrease the absorption of lead (Barton *et al.*, 1981). In their studies on humans Watson *et al.* (1980) showed that iron-deficient human subjects absorbed two to three times more lead than normal subjects when given as a carrier-free tracer dose of lead-203. In these subjects there was a highly significant linear relationship between the percentage oral iron absorption and the percentage oral absorption of lead. It was estimated that, taking into account the conditions of the experiment, iron-deficient subjects can absorb around 24 per cent of dietary lead intake as compared to the normal absorption of around 10 per cent.

Other Materials.   There is a catalogue of other substances that can influence the absorption of lead. In general substances influencing the intestinal barrier such as ethanol will increase lead absorption (Mahaffey *et al.*, 1974). Substances that increase lead solubility will also increase absorption. Examples of this are solubilisation with acids such as ascorbic or citric acid, or combination with compounds such as amino acids (Conrad and Barton, 1978), although the effects of amino acids upon absorption are age related and related to the type of amino acid involved (Quarterman *et al.*, 1980) and to the presence of chelating agents (Jugo *et al.*, 1975). Compounds such as tannic acid and thiamine have been reported to exert protective effects on animals given dietary lead. This may relate to their ability to bind heavy metals and thus enhance their excretion or alternatively like amino acids to alter their tissue distribution (Barton *et al.*, 1981; Peaslee and Einhellig, 1977). In man the use of alginates as food additives has been shown to have no effect on lead absorption whereas small but significant increases in absorption were found in rats (Harrison *et al.*, 1969). Other major dietary components likely to influence absorption are carbohydrates, which would appear to have little effect, lipids which increase lead uptake (Barltrop and Khoo, 1976) and dietary proteins which have complex effects but in general lower dietary lead absorption (Quarterman *et al.*, 1978). The effects of lipids have been associated with increased concentration of phospholipid and ultimately with stimulation of bile flow which adds phospholipid and bile salts to gut lumen contents and thus enhances absorption (Quarterman *et al.*, 1977).

Alteration of Toxicity

Toxicity following absorption can also be affected by concentrations of dietary compounds. Thawley *et al.* (1977) found that toxic concentrations of other metals such as zinc or cadmium caused a marked diminution in the toxic effects of lead such as reticulocytosis and diminution in the activity of amino laevulinic acid (ALA) dehydratase (Meredith *et al.*, 1977a). High dietary zinc concentrations will diminish lead levels in all tissues, a role that is reversed in zinc deficiency, which would suggest that there is a protective role for zinc in lead toxicity (Cerklewski and Forbes, 1976; El-Gazzar *et al.*, 1978; Bushnell and Levin, 1983). Similar effects have been observed for aluminium (Meredith *et al.*, 1977a). Selenium is another element exhibiting antagonistic toxic effects.

At toxic concentrations lead and selenium result in normal activities of ALA dehydratase and cytochrome P450 activity in rats (Cerklewski and Forbes, 1976; Rastogi *et al.*, 1976). A similar positive correlation has been reported between concentrations of vitamin E and tissue lead concentrations (Sleet and Soares, 1978) and indeed other vitamins such as thiamine are diminished by increased concentrations of lead (Tokarski and Reio, 1978) whilst other substances such as ascorbic acid and other lead binding agents such as cysteine can decrease lead toxicity by increasing its excretion (McNiff *et al.*, 1978). The effects of vitamin D have already been discussed and it should be noted that when vitamin D is administered blood lead concentrations in animals decrease, this is associated with decreased loss of lead from bone (Sobel and Burger, 1955).

Renal accumulation of lead is increased when parathyroid hormone is administered to rats and in consequence there is an increased possibility of toxic effects on the kidney(Mouw *et al.*, 1978). These effects are attributed to increased formation of insoluble lead phosphate in the kidney cells although they may also have been attributed to changes in tubular reabsorption in the kidney. In fact, Quarterman *et al.* (1977) found increased lead content in the kidneys of castrated rams but surprisingly, greater mortality in normal animals. The results implied that hormonal effects will also influence the absorption and excretion of lead (Kostial *et al.*, 1974). Sulphate additions to diet diminished the toxic effects of lead which was attributed to the formation of insoluble lead phosphates during rumen digestion which by binding lead lowered its retention.

Excretion

Dietary components also influence retention by altering rates of excretion of lead from the body. Although increased calcium levels decreased loss of lead, vitamin D increases its loss (Barton *et al.*, 1980) whereas iron does not appear to influence the excretion at all (Barton *et al.*, 1978b). The other therapeutic compounds most commonly implicated in the enhanced clearance of lead in the body are chelating agents. Compounds such as penicillamine and ethylene diaminotetra-acetic acid (EDTA) are commonly used in the treatment of lead poisoning (Goldberg *et al.*, 1963). They function by increasing the urinary excretion of lead as its chelated complex. Penicillamine is readily absorbed from the gastrointestinal tract and can be given orally whereas EDTA is poorly absorbed and is generally given by intravenous injection. Such enhancement of urinary excretion of lead is common to all chelating agents. These are increasingly found as components of foods either as natural compounds or food additives (Furia, 1968). Acidic compounds, such as citric acid or ascorbic acid, have more equivocal results. In both cases these compounds have such rapid rates of metabolism that following absorption they can have little or no effect on subsequent urinary excretion of lead. Where, however, blockade of the citric acid cycle takes place as with monofluoroacetic acid modest doses of sodium citrate seem to provide animals with protection against lead poisoning (Schubert and Lindenbaum, 1960).

An Example — Milk.   In general, therefore, the difficulty in assessing the potential effects of components of diet and diet on lead absorption and excretion is evident (Moore, 1979; Mahaffey, 1980). Even when viewed individually it is not always clear whether the net effect of a single dietary component will be beneficial or otherwise. Calcium which would appear to be a useful compound in the prophylaxis of lead poisoning can produce only small changes in the blood lead status of lead workers (Moore *et al.*, 1978b). The whole problem is perhaps best exemplified by the example of milk as a whole food in diet. There are a number of different components in milk, some of which, like lactose, will *increase* lead absorption (Bushnell and Deluca, 1981) whilst others, like calcium, lower absorption. Some components will raise or lower the toxic effects following absorption and finally there are some which increase and some which will cause a diminution in the excretion of absorbed lead. The net effect might either be an enhancement or diminution in lead absorption with milk depending on the nutritional status of each specific subject (Stephens and Waldron, 1975; Bell and Spickett, 1981). The only conclusion that one can reasonably arrive at, therefore, is that only in the circumstance where a dietary component is found in great excess or great deficiency, will one be able to divine the likely outcome in terms of lead toxicity.

Tissue Lead Uptake

The actual concentrations of lead in human tissues have been examined carefully by a number of authors. Perhaps the most extensive studies were carried out by Barry (1975, 1981) who examined the concentrations of lead in the tissues of adults and children in post-mortem studies. Similar work was carried out by Schroeder and Tipton (1968) and Gross *et al.* (1975). The net information from these studies is that lead is stored principally in bone in the body. This accumulation begins in fetal life, because the placenta does not limit transfer of lead from mother to the fetus (Moore, 1980) and continues until death. The total body burden of lead in adults can be as high as 200 mg in men but is generally lower in women (Horiuchi *et al.*, 1959). This means that about 94-95 per cent of the total body burden of lead is in the bones. There are some variations however, in bone lead concentrations. Rib concentrations tend to reach a maximum between the ages of 60-70 years as do vertebrae whilst the long bones continue to accumulate lead until death, a feature in common with the soft tissues (Table 5.1).

Lead in Bone

It is perhaps appropriate then at this stage to consider just how lead is taken up into bone and the uses of this. That lead is taken up in relatively large quantities is without question. Furthermore it is taken up rapidly, as has been shown in some studies where lead-203 has been suggested as a potential radionucleide for skeletal imaging (Rao and Goodwin, 1973). It has also been used as a

Table 5.1: Concentrations of Lead in Humans

Estimated for man 30 years environmental exposure

Tissue	Range of concentrations
Whole body	62-140 mg
Aorta	27-150 µg/g ash
Blood	2-30 µg/100 ml whole blood
Bone (long)	26-89 µg/g ash
Brain	5-14 µg/g ash
Hair	2-100 µg/g
Kidney	36-98 µg/g ash
Liver	59-160 µg/g ash
Teeth	8-100 µg/g ash

means of assessing 'so called' natural concentrations of lead in humans. To do this, bone lead measurements have been made on skeletal remains in Nubia and Peru from time periods before the industrial use of lead (Grandjean *et al.*, 1979; Erickson *et al.*, 1979). These studies appear to show a greater than 10-fold increase in bone lead concentrations when compared with contemporary values in bone. In some cases evidence of lead poisoning has been found in ancient remains (Shapiro *et al.*, 1980; Aufderheide *et al.*, 1981). There has, however, been some criticism of this technique of evaluation since subsequent studies have shown that the concentrations of lead in such bones are greatest at the bone surface. In England it was found that there was a significant correlation between concentrations of lead in bone and soils taken from the same grave (Barry and Connelly, 1981; Waldron, 1982) suggesting very strongly that there had been exchange of lead between soil and bones. In lead poisoning, since bone is the seat of deposition, one finds that particularly the growing ends of long bones in children, are affected. This shows up as a line of dense material on X-ray (Figure 5.4) but does not interfere with growth or integrity.

Teeth

Bone biopsies are, in any case, extremely difficult to obtain in living human beings. Another form of bone biopsy is, however, readily available mainly in children, but also in adults, and that is from teeth lost at the time of abscission of primary dentition or because of extraction for caries. This type of analysis has attracted considerable interest in recent years and work in the USA and other areas of the world showed that the lead content of deciduous teeth of children living in urban areas, was greater than those living in suburban or rural areas (Needleman *et al.*, 1972; Stewart, 1974; Rytoma and Tuompo, 1974; Kaneko *et al.*, 1974; Shapiro *et al.*, 1975; Lockeretz, 1975; Stack *et al.*, 1975, 1976; Fosse *et al.*, 1978). Thus dentition, like bone, is a good indicator of past exposure to lead.

Such lead accumulation is dose related and permanent within the tooth (Strehlow, 1972). Although most tooth lead would appear to be laid down from the circulation during formation and eruption, there is a possibility that deposition on the surface can occur directly in the mouth. The work of Steadman *et al.* (1959) does not support this. Since tooth lead is laid down continuously

Figure 5.4: Features of Lead Poisoning. The upper radiograph
shows the electron-dense line found in the bone, and in the lower
the microscope appearance of the ring sideroblast in bone
marrow is shown

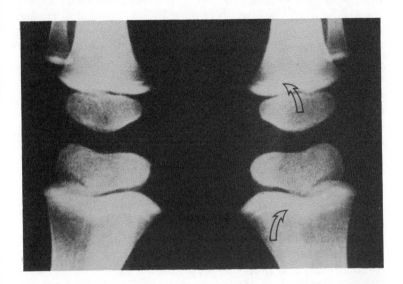

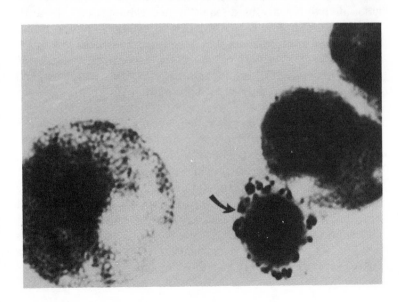

concentrations are age related (Pfrieme, 1934; Needleman *et al.*, 1974; Stewart, 1974; Wilkinson and Palmer, 1975). Such age-related rises reach a plateau towards the end of the third decade (Holtzman *et al.*, 1968). The highest concentrations of lead within teeth have been identified as lying within the circumpulpal dentine zone (Pfrieme, 1934; Shapiro *et al.*, 1973, 1975) although enamel concentrations are greater than dentine (Malik and Fremlin, 1974) and concentrations have been found to vary across the enamel (Brudevold and Steadman, 1956). Interestingly, children with high enamel lead concentrations have a higher caries score than children with low enamel lead (Brudevold *et al.*, 1977). Tooth lead also varies considerably with tooth type (Strehlow, 1972; Lockeretz, 1975; Mackie *et al.*, 1977; Delves *et al.*, 1982) and lead concentration in the root portion of the tooth tends to be higher than that in the crown (Pinchin *et al.*, 1978; Delves *et al.*, 1982). This is probably related to the chronology of root resorption especially of deciduous teeth. Although dentine lead content increases with age (Al-Naimi *et al.*, 1980) there is no equivalent rise in enamel which is consistent with the endogenous rather than exogenous accumulation of lead in teeth in different exposure situations (Steenhout and Pourtois, 1981).

Tooth lead concentrations vary with the degree of exposure. However, tooth lead levels in urban industrial situations are associated with generalised exposure and cannot usually be attributed to one specific source (Mackie *et al.*, 1977) although in a limited number of instances they have been linked with lead smelters (Stack *et al*, 1975), urban water exposure (Moore *et al*, 1978a), pica (De la Burdé and Shapiro, 1975; Joselow and Bogden, 1977) and lead paint (Shapiro *et al.*, 1975).

Despite this it has been suggested that because of considerable variation in tooth lead concentrations even in the same mouth and tooth type, the value of tooth lead measurement might be questioned (Delves *et al.*, 1982). The fact remains, however, that imperfect as it might be, it provides a good measure of long-term integrated exposure to lead and as such, together with other imperfect measures of lead exposure, such as lead in blood, will probably continue to be used to assess exposure. The mean concentration of lead in teeth expressed on a dry weight basis is between 4.1 and 5.6 µg/g for children living within cities in the UK which is slightly lower than those reported in the USA.

Figure 5.5: The Blue Line — a Deposition of Lead Sulphide at the Gingival Margin Associated With Poor Dental Hygiene, As Well As With Lead Poisoning

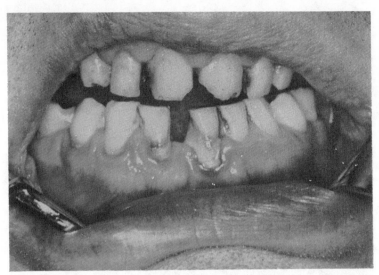

The Blue Line. A common feature of lead poisoning especially where there is poor dental hygiene is the formation of the so called Burtonian blue line at the gingival margin. Microscopic studies of such lines show that there is both extra- and intracellular deposition of lead-containing material. The extracellular lead is deposited between the collagen fibres and around the blood vessels of the dermal and epidermal junction whilst intracellular lead is found within the membrane-bound microsomes and on the cytoplasmic and mitochondrial membrane. This formation of the lead line is thought to be due to the precipitation of lead-sulphur compounds formed by the action of sulpho-bacteria on lead in the gingival fluid (Honigsmann *et al.*, 1974) (Figure 5.5).

Other Tissues

Specific measurements have been made of lead concentrations in other tissues. In the lungs, for instance, greater concentrations were found in segments of the upper lobe and the concentrations in the regional lymph nodes were greater than those in the lung segments (Mylius and Ophus, 1977). This is a pointer to the considerable variations within tissues as well as the differences found

Figure 5.6: The Distribution (Percentage) of Lead in the Various Components of Blood

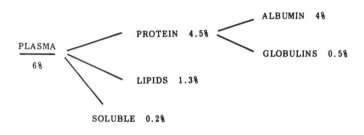

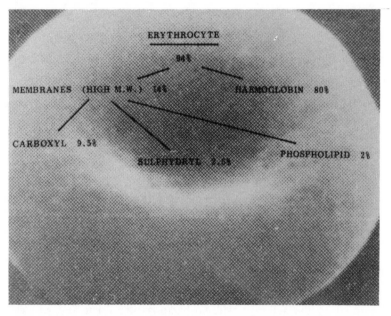

between tissues. Of body fluids, blood lead has been the one most examined because it is the most reliable and available source of biopsy material from humans. Other body fluids have however been examined. Semen and sweat have been found to have lead concentrations less than that in blood but to show relationship with blood lead levels, as does breast milk (Figure 5.6) (Hohnadel *et al.*, 1973; Plechaty *et al.*, 1977). In general the concentration of lead in body fluids tends to be less than that of blood. In blood, lead is associated principally with the red cells. The concentration in blood plasma is less than one tenth of that in the red blood cells, similar to the concentration in milk. Thus subjects with variable degrees of lead poisoning have plasma lead levels which are proportionately much lower (Rosen *et al.*, 1974).

Distribution

The Erythrocyte

The red cell is in fact the principal transport component of lead from the gut or the lungs to the various other tissues in the body and it is therefore of considerable importance how the lead is bound to the blood and whether such bound lead can influence the physiological characteristics of blood in its primary capacity as an oxygen transport mechanism. The earliest studies showed that lead is bound to the red blood cell (Clarkson and Kench, 1958; Barltrop and Smith, 1971). More recently, lead within the red blood cell was found to be bound primarily to haemoglobin. This uptake by the erythroctye can be inhibited by iron (Kaplan *et al.*, 1976). Since lead cannot be dialysed from the red cell, it is probable that an insoluble lead-haemoglobin complex is formed (Clarkson and Kench, 1958; Ong and Lee, 1980b). Although lead will bind to a number of proteins, its strongest binding within the blood and with the red cell is to haemoglobin with a particular affinity for fetal haemoglobin (HbF) (Ong and Lee, 1980b). About 80 per cent of lead in blood is bound in this way (Figure 5.6). The distribution here provides an interesting microcosm of the processes of binding and distribution within other soft tissues. In this respect, it is of interest that other than the binding to haemoglobin the strongest binding components are the proteins with very limited quantities associated with lipid. Since so much lead is bound to haemoglobin, the strength of binding will be an important determinant of biological effect since only that part of the lead in the blood which is free is available for transport to other organs or indeed to have toxic effects upon other biochemical systems within the red cell.

Ligand Binding

It has previously been generally accepted that lead will bind preferentially to sulphydryl groups. Examination of the blood does not confirm this supposition. Sulphydryl groups do play a role in the binding of lead to globins but the major binding ligands are carboxyl groups. This may partly explain the mechanisms by which lead is capable of inhibiting the activity of sodium/potassium dependent ATPase within the red cell. Membrane carboxyl groups are involved in the formation of an intermediate for this enzyme and if lead combines with such carboxyl groups at the active site the enzyme will be inhibited. Red cell membrane studies using calcium-45 indicate that calcium is bound to the same fraction of membrane proteins as lead and it is therefore possible that lead and calcium will compete for the same binding sites upon the erythrocyte membrane (Ong, 1980; Ong and Lee, 1980c).

The basophilic stippling (Figure 5.7) found in cells from patients with lead poisoning is due in part at least to changes in the ribosomes. This change is not specific to lead poisoning and indeed is found in haemolytic anaemias, leukaemia and alcoholism. The stippling is caused by deposition of altered cytoplasmic elements including ribosomal RNA and mitochondrial fragments (Bessis and Jensen, 1965). Similarly the ring sideroblast (Figure 5.4) which is found in lead poisoning is more commonly found following alcoholic intoxication (Moore *et al.*, 1983). As a consequence of the changes that lead causes to the red cell there is considerable

Figure 5.7: The Stippled Basophil Found in Lead Poisoning

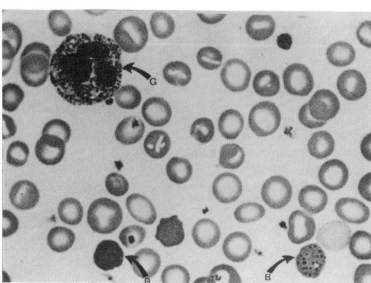

shortening of the red cell life span. This is probably due to a direct toxic effect upon the cell membrane (Moore and Goldberg, 1983).

Distribution in Other Tissues — Excretion

The actual distribution of lead in other tissues would seem to suggest that it is bound to intracellular organelles (Barltrop *et al.*, 1971; Moore, 1975) and some workers have suggested a preference for binding to the mitochondrion (Castellino and Aloj, 1969). In general lead taken up by the organs shows that the kidney has the greatest percentage uptake followed by the liver and then other soft tissues such as heart and brain (Table 5.1). This preference for the kidney may be reflected in the fact that renal excretion is the principal means by which the body rids itself of this metal (Waldron and Stofen, 1974). This urinary clearance of lead is essentially through glomerular filtration although the actual form of the excreted lead is not known (Vostal, 1966; WHO, 1977). It is for these reasons that urinary lead concentrations have been used to estimate lead exposure especially in industry. It has been found, however, that urinary lead concentrations show very large variations and are often difficult to analyse because of matrix interference. This also applies to the measurement of urinary lead in chelation tests where EDTA is given by injection and the amount of chelatable lead excreted measured. There are problems also in obtaining appropriate samples for this test and for that reason people have settled generally on the use of blood lead as a measure of current exposure. Chelatable lead however is the best indicator of lead concentrations since it provides a measurement of the 'rapid-exchange' pool of lead within the soft tissues of the body (Zielhuis, 1975; Alessio *et al.*, 1979). The use of hair lead concentrations has been suggested as a means of measurement of longer-term exposure to this metal. Measurement of hair lead suffers greatly from the rapid and irreversible adsorption of the metal onto the surfaces of the hair by topical contamination. This obviously does not reflect the clearance of endogenous lead in the hair (Renshaw *et al.*, 1972; Klevay and Hyg, 1973).

Experimental Studies in Humans

The first and most famous studies of lead uptake by humans were carried out by Robert Kehoe between 1937 and 1972. His studies concentrated on the balance of lead in the human body following dietary supplementation at different levels between 300 and 3000 µg/day over extended time periods. In the first of these studies he concluded that although there was considerable variability in the amount of lead taken in by the body, around 10 per cent of lead in the diet would be absorbed and retained (Kehoe, 1961; Kehoe *et al.*, 1943) effectively showing that the bodily balance of lead increased by 0.133 µg/day for every µg of lead in the diet (Gross, 1981). Subsequent experiments using radioactive lead as a tracer have generally confirmed these findings and have shown in addition that the quantity of food already in the gut as well as the dietary parameters described previously can play a considerable role in the actual quantity of lead absorbed (Rabinowitz *et al.*, 1973, 1980; Hursh and Suomela, 1968; Blake, 1976; Moore *et al.*, 1979) which is also influenced by age (Ziegler *et al.*, 1978). Indeed on very low dietary intakes of lead the children are in negative balance.

The Curvilinear Relationship

From their studies Chamberlain *et al.* (1978) predicted that the increase in blood lead for every microgram of lead in the diet would be 36 ng/100 ml. These calculations were made on the basis of a linear relationship between exposure and absorption. There is more than sufficient evidence at the present time to show that this is not the case. For example, acquisition of tolerance to lead especially where higher levels of exposure are experienced over long periods of time has been found and The Duplicate Diet Studies carried out in the UK (DOE, 1982; Sherlock *et al.*, 1982; Lacey· *et al.*, 1985) and the study of lead uptake from water supplies have shown non-linear relationships (Moore *et al.*, 1977) (Figure 5.2). The relationship between exposure and blood lead concentrations and therefore presumably also bodily lead levels is curvilinear with the rate of increase at lower levels of exposure being much greater than the rate of increase at higher levels of exposure. The existence of this curvilinear relationship probably explains why research studies cannot fully account for blood lead concentrations found in the general population. It is true to say, however, that within the constraints of normal ranges of exposure to lead, the reported results are satisfactorily explained on the basis of linear relationship (Lacey *et al.*, in press).

This curvilinear relationship also probably applies to exposure from the air although as yet it has not been conclusively demonstrated. The fate of inhaled lead remains a matter of conjecture. A proportion is certainly deposited in the upper respiratory tract and shifted by ciliary action to the throat where it is swallowed. Lead that gets to the lower part of the lung is probably solubilised and rapidly absorbed. The reported rate of increase in blood lead following exposure to lead in the air is very variable. This rate is termed α being defined as the increase in $\mu g/100$ ml of blood lead for every increase of 1 $\mu g/m^3$ of lead in air. Kehoe's experiments estimated this as being as low as 0.57 whereas Rabinowitz *et al.* (1973) and Chamberlain *et al.* (1975) gave values of 1.2. O'Brien *et al.* (1980) estimated the value as 1.7 and the highest reported figure lies somewhat in excess of 2 (Chamberlain *et al.*, 1978). Doubts remain about the most appropriate value for this unit. As with food, the evidence must be that as the air lead concentrations rise so the values of α fall (Hammond *et al.*, 1979). In exposure chamber studies, Coulston *et al.* (1972) showed that at an exposure level of 10.9 $\mu g/m^3$ blood lead levels rose by 18 $\mu g/100$ ml giving a value of absorption of 1.65, similar to those proposed previously. Specific studies of the respiratory absorption of lead have been reported using lead-212 which showed that the half-life for absorption from airways ranged between 6 and 12 hours (Hursh and Mercer, 1970). Subsequent experiments showed similar biological half-life of around 14 hours with around 25 per cent deposition in the lung (Morrow *et al.*, 1980), all of which would be absorbed. All of these figures are of course calculated for adults. For children experimental studies are unjustifiably risky. It has been calculated, however, that for a 10-year-old child percentage retention of small particles in the air will be greater than that in adults and that 70 per cent of inhaled lead will be deposited in the respiratory tract of children and all will be absorbed (DHSS, 1980).

Models of Exposure, Retention and Excretion

From the available information that has by now accrued on this subject, many authors have now attempted to fit kinetic models relating these various parameters. The usual approach has been to formulate a multicompartmental model where each compartment represents an organ or a system in which the lead is assumed to have a constant composition at equilibrium. As will be appreciated the composition of lead within a given tissue is far from constant.

Figure 5.8: A Model of Lead Absorption, Distribution and Excretion

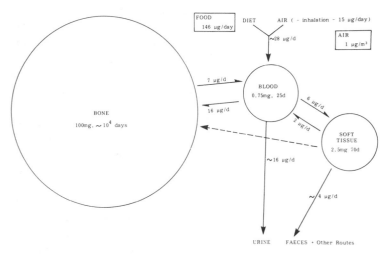

However, it is often possible to use this technique where, during continuous input of lead, the spatial distribution within the organ remains constant with time.

The model most commonly relied upon is similar to that proposed by Rabinowitz *et al.* (1976) which uses three compartments. There is a central compartment approximating to the blood with a soft tissue and bone compartment dependent on a dynamic equilibrium in which lead input to the blood equilibrates with time into the other two compartments (Figure 5.8). This type of model was further developed to give five compartments in which the additional two compartments comprise lungs and the digestive tract (Batschlet *et al.*, 1979), which is rather different to the model proposed by Bernard (1977) in which there are three soft tissue compartments or that of Blake (1980) which proposed no less than 25 compartments to cover all eventualities of tissue distribution. In a comparison of some of these models Marcus (1979) showed that at least two bone compartments would be needed to cover satisfactorily all of the requirements of lead exposure, uptake and distribution. The complexity of this can be readily appreciated from the exposure commitment techniques formulated by O'Brien (1979) to create a mathematical model for exposure to lead.

In general by increasing the complexity of the model by using greater and greater numbers of compartments, parameters and variables it becomes possible to represent the physical system more exactly. In practice it is more acceptable to limit the number of compartments in order to simplify and thus make more comprehensible the physical characteristics of the system. The real problem in making such models for lead is that all the mathematics used to date have assumed that the effects follow linear relationships. This is not so for the reasons stated previously. However, within the constraint of a limited exposure level range, a linear system is a reasonable approximation.

Acute and Chronic Exposure.   Two distinct situations exist in the assessment of exposure to lead. There is acute exposure and chronic exposure. Acute exposure corresponds to a person who has become lead poisoned following excessive exposure to lead over a short period of time. The worker who has recently entered into lead industry approximates to this situation; it is typified by the experimental model in which a single dose of lead is administered intravenously and the changes in tissue distributions followed over time.

Chronic exposure is exemplified by the pattern of consistent exposure to elevated levels of lead over long periods of time, as is found in environmental exposure to sources of lead, such as excessive lead in drinking water, or equally, exposure of workers in the lead industry to greater than normal concentrations of lead in their working environment over long periods of time. Such exposure will be through both pulmonary and gastrointestinal absorption. The rates of absorption by these two routes differ but following retention the actual handling of the absorbed lead will be similar.

Absorbed lead can enter effectively into three different compartments in the body corresponding to the various compartments in the models described previously. There is the short-term transport compartment — the blood; the longer-term intermediate storage compartment — the soft tissues; and finally the long-term, long half-life and very large storage compartment found in bone. Of these three compartments, the first two — blood and soft tissues — will reach a dynamic equilibrium following constant exposure after a relatively short period of time with the half-life of lead in blood being about 60 days. It is unlikely, however, that the bone storage compartment ever truly reaches equilibrium especially since some bone lead may be mobilised in certain conditions such as stress (Waldron and Stofen, 1974). The absorbed lead may then be excreted either in the urine or in the faeces, and a small amount will also be lost by exfoliation of the surface layer of the skin and shedding of hair. Different workers have given various values for the distribution of such excreted lead between urine and faeces. Generally, however, faecal lead concentrations are very much higher than urinary lead concentrations, principally because most ingested lead is not absorbed and passes directly through the gastrointestinal tract to be excreted. This makes endogenous faecal excretion difficult to measure, since although most absorbed lead is excreted in the urine, some is excreted in the faeces.

Absorption.   There are various unsatisfactory features when one assesses absorption of lead from both the gut and the lungs in the general steady-state condition and in the extrapolation from environmental to industrial levels of exposure. One such feature is that the balance between pulmonary and gastrointestinal absorption is not known. Pulmonary absorption will give a rise of 1-2 $\mu g/100$ ml of blood lead for every 1 $\mu g/m^3$ Pb in the air. This will rise to 2.6 mg/100 ml when one takes into consideration the storage lead component (Chamberlain *et al.*, 1978). This is a much greater figure than would normally be found for gastrointestinal absorption where a mean figure of around 10-20 per cent absorption in environmental circumstances is probably appropriate.

Excretion.   In carrying out calculations on lead absorption and excretion, it is necessary to make a number of assumptions. First, one must decide upon the type of model being dealt with — whether a steady-state model in equilibrium or an acute dosage model. One must assume in calculating exposure levels that all the lead taken in is bioavailable and may be absorbed. This assumption is patently untrue since by no means all lead ingested or inhaled is available for absorption. Excreted lead in faeces must be calculated from the ratio of endogenous faecal to urinary excretion. Since most studies measuring the distribution between urine and faeces are based on relatively low levels of exposure, the figures on distribution used in any calculations in the industrial situation assume that the ratio between urinary and faecal excretion remains the same regardless of the quantity of lead absorbed, which again over-simplifies the probable relationship.

In the very simplest situation, one can assume that when exposure is constant or relatively constant and a form of equilibrium has been reached, then all material absorbed must be balanced by an equal quantity of lead excreted which will be the sum of urinary and faecal excretion. Only the earliest balance studies, carried out by Kehoe (1961) measured the total concentrations of lead in faeces. Subsequent work has concentrated upon the quantity of lead found in urine. It is therefore necessary to calculate total absorption on the basis of models which calculate the ratio between urinary and faecal excretion. Many different figures have been given for this and the ones used here (0.23, 0.05) are those calculated from intravenous dosage data, using lead-203 in normal humans (Moore *et al.*, 1979).

Storage. In the steady-state lead exposure situation, there is a further component which complicates any calculations. That is, stored lead, which is that part of absorbed lead not excreted but stored in bone. This is relatively constant and stable with a long half-life which may be measured in years as compared with the half-life of lead in blood of about one month (Rabinowitz *et al.*, 1976). Thus, during a life-time of exposure, there is a daily long-term storage of about 9 μg of lead in non-occupationally exposed persons (Barry, 1975). This quantity of lead represents transfer from both the blood and the soft tissue compartments. This storage component is generally not bioavailable but does account for the differences between the rates of absorption and excretion found in many studies. Although accurate figures on likely storage in lead workers is not available, one can reasonably assume that the distribution of lead is similar in occupational and environmental exposure subjects, since both have similar distribution of lead in bone and soft tissues (Barry, 1975).

Computer-Model. The three-compartment model to be used is shown in Figure 5.8. The rate constants between each of the compartments are open to conjecture. This model includes a storage component giving a net daily accumulation of around 9 μg of lead in bone. The computer model can be applied in two ways: first a single (100 per cent) dose of lead is given and the changes in concentration followed over a long time period. This demonstrates that in the acute dose situation, blood concentrations of lead rise rapidly, after which there is a fairly rapid increase in soft tissue concentrations and excretion. There is a very much slower, and lesser increase, in the total accumulation in bone.

The alternative situation is where there is a constant input of single doses over a long period of time, like the chronic exposure situation and similar to environmental overexposure. Where doses were administered over 20 weeks equilibrium was not achieved.

Calculations of Exposure

Industrial Exposure

Excretion.   Cooper and Gaffey (1975) and (1976) calculated that, for 1550 workers, 1053 in battery plants and 497 in smelters, the mean urinary lead (PbU) was 129.7 μg/l in battery plants and 173.2 μg/l in smelters. If one assumes that these workers are populations in equilibrium and that the volume of urine excreted daily by heavy manual workers is at the upper end of the population normal, that is 1600 ml, then the quantity of lead excreted in urine (U) by battery plant workers will be 194.55 μg/day and in smelter plant workers, 259.8 μg/day. Faecal excretion (F) is then calculated from the ratio of 0.23 mentioned previously.
Then

$$\text{Total excreted lead (PbE)} = F + U$$
$$= 0.23\,U + U$$

In battery plants, this will give a figure of 239.3 μg/day and in smelters, a figure of 319.5 μg/day. This assumes that other excretory routes, such as sweat, desquamation of the skin and hair, are small and may be neglected. In excess exposure situations, the increased urinary clearance of lead is given by the equation:

$$\text{renal clearance} = \frac{\text{the amount of lead excreted in urine/h}}{\text{the amount/g of blood}}$$

There is no evidence to date to show whether or not there is an equivalent rise in the quantity of lead cleared in faeces (i.e. whether or not the ratio of faecal to urinary excretion remains constant). The renal clearance has been calculated in normal subjects to be around 4.5 g/h.
The total absorbed lead must then be the sum of the total excretion and that component of absorbed lead that goes into

long-term storage in bone, thus:

Total daily absorbed lead (PbT) = PbE + storage

= 395 µg/day

(for smelter workers)

The storage component is calculated in this case from the studies of Kehoe, (1961). In normal subjects, Barry (1975) found that 9 µg day of absorbed lead went into long-term storage in bone, but this figure is certainly too small for workers in the lead industry in whom others have calculated that 0.4 per cent of the uptake will be stored. The figure given by Kehoe (1961) of around 76 µg/day is used here and it is probable that figures in excess of this will be accurate in long-term lead workers.

If one assigns a 50 per cent distribution to gastrointestinal and pulmonary exposure vectors, then:

Total lead exposure = F_1 × (gastrointestinal uptake of lead)
+ F_2 × (pulmonary intake of lead)

where F_1 and F_2 are factors determining the rates of absorption of lead from these two organs. F_1 will be around 5.52 according to a 18.1 per cent uptake from the gut (Blake, 1976; Chamberlain *et al.*, 1978; Moore *et al.*, 1979) and F_2 around 2 according to a 50 per cent absorption from the lungs. In sum therefore, the total exposure to lead can be calculated from the total of absorbed lead in smelter workers as equal to:

Total exposure to lead = 5.52 × 197.7 + 2.0 × 197.7
= 1487.1 µg/day

This figure is a gross oversimplification since by no means all of the industrial lead exposure will be bioavailable and since many assumptions have been made regarding the distribution and allocation to both absorptive and excretory routes. If the lead bioavailable for absorption for instance was taken in totally through the lungs, then the exposure figure could be as low as 791 µg/day and if absorbed totally through the gut, could be as high as 2183.16 µg/day. In addition, some lead in both circumstances is not readily bioavailable which makes even the higher of these figures an underestimate.

Blood. These problems of transferral from excretory figures are seen even more clearly in consideration of the rate of increase of blood lead with respect to gastrointestinal absorption of lead. If one defines the rate of increase in blood lead following oral intake of lead as μg% increase/100 μg oral lead/day, (μg%/d) then for a mean gastrointestinal absorption of 18 per cent, the rate of change of blood lead will be 3.6 μg%/d. Practical experience has shown that this figure is almost certainly too high but it must be borne in mind that it is dose dependent. Increased exposure rates almost certainly mean lowered absorption of lead from the gastrointestinal tract as a homeostatic protective mechanism. A similar figure can be calculated for pulmonary exposure to lead, that is, calculating the rate of increase of blood lead with respect to the rate of increase in air lead, being expressed as μg/100 ml increase/ m^3 lead in air (μg %/m^3) (where air lead exposure is the 24 hour exposure mean the so called 'α' unit first calculated as 1.2 but later corrected to 2.6 (Chamberlain *et al.*, 1978) which corresponds to the calculated epidemiological figures (Tsuchiya *et al.*, 1975).

Similar therefore to the calculation carried out on the urinary data, it is possible to calculate lead workers' exposure from the available blood data. Industrial blood lead values reach plateau levels after about one month's exposure indicating that dynamic equilibrium has been reached. The mean concentration given by Cooper (1976) is 79.7 μg% for smelter workers. As with the urinary data, the assumption made is that each of these workers is in equilibrium in his working environment. This is a reasonable assumption since this figure is a mean of a very large number of measurements. If it is accepted, that a normal urban male subject is exposed to lead such that his blood lead concentration will reach a mean value of 15 μg%, then any blood lead in excess of this value must be due to the industrial exposure. Thus the excess exposure in the smelter workers accounts for 64.7 μg% of the total blood lead value.

It may be calculated that 3.2 μg% of blood lead accrues for every 100 μg of lead in the daily diet (Rabinowitz *et al.*, 1976). This then means that around 2000 μg of lead can be associated with gastrointestinal exposure and 500 μg/day for exposure through the lungs (Table 5.2). The calculated air lead exposure of 24 μg/m^3 is within the range of air lead concentrations found in industrial circumstances. The total exposure to lead of the workers is a sum of this industrial exposure and the domestic exposure, i.e.:

Table 5.2: Industrial Exposure

Changes of blood lead concentration following gastrointestinal and pulmonary lead exposure
Normal blood lead 15 μg%
Smelter workers blood lead (mean) 79.7 μg%
Increase in blood lead over normal 64.7 μg%
(assessed to be exclusively due to industrial exposure)

1. *Oral intake*
If one assumes that PbB/Pb ingested = 3.2 μg%/100 μg/day
then a rise in PbB of 64.7 μg% is equivalent to oral exposure of 2021 μg/day

2. *Pulmonary intake*
If one calculates PbB/Pb air = 2.6 μg%/m³ (Chamberlain *et al.*, 1978)
then a rise in PbB of 64.7 μg% is equivalent to pulmonary exposure of 24.9 μg/m³
If 20 m³ air is breathed daily, at that rate = pulmonary exposure of 498 μg/day

---

Total exposure = industrial exposure
    + domestic exposure taken from Table 5.3

= 1259 1 (for 50 per cent pulmonary and GI exposure
    Table 5.2 + 161

= 1420 μg/day

This figure is very similar to the calculated excretion figure. Potential sources of error are (1) distribution between gut and lungs; (2) the figures for PbB and (3) the volume of air breathed may be very much greater than 20 m³ in industrial workers.

Urban Environmental Exposure

In Table 5.3, a possible balance scheme is given for an adult white male, aged 30, social class 3, weight 70 kg in a large city in the United Kingdom who smokes 20 cigarettes per day and drinks moderate quantities of beer. In this, various assumptions are made. Blood volume is taken as 5 litres. Mean air lead is taken as 1 μg/m³ for 24 h exposure, which is high even for the centre of cities, such as Birmingham, Bristol and London (Lawther *et al.*, 1973; Archer and Barratt, 1976; Day *et al.*, 1977; DHSS, 1980). In the calculations, the daily intake of air has been calculated as 15 m³/day and lung absorption as 40 per cent. The percentage absorption from air of 21.5 per cent is in good agreement with experimental studies (Facchetti *et al.*, 1982). For this subject, alimentary

Table 5.3: Uptake and Excretion of Lead by Adult Male in Urban Britain

Blood lead	15 μg/dl
Intake in food and drink	146 μg/day
Air lead (24 h average)	1 μg/m³
Absorption	
% absorption by gut	15%
Uptake of lead from GI tract	21.9 μg/day
Uptake from lungs (40% is absorbed)	6.0 μg/day
Total uptake	27.9 μg/day
Excretion	
Urinary excretion	16 μg/day
Endogenous faecal excretion	3.7 μg/day
(based on mean F/U ratio of 0.23)	
Total excretion	19.7 μg/day
Residue — Storage — Bone	8.2 μg/day

absorption of lead is taken as 21.9 μg/day, calculated from a 15 per cent absorption from the gut and intake level of 146 μg/day (DHSS, 1980). The mean blood lead level of 15 μg% is typical of median figures found in many urban industrial areas of the United Kingdom (DOE, 1983). The calculations also take into account that IRCP reference man has a total lead burden of 120 mg (IRCP, 1975) and that urinary excretion of lead is 16 μg/day (Harrison and Laxen, 1981). With the faecal to urinary excretion ratios taken as 0.23, endogenous faecal excretion is 3.7 μg/day, leaving a net positive balance of 8.2 μg/day, which is similar to the measured 9 μg/day of lead stored in bone (Barry, 1975).

Where there is increased exposure due to, for example, increased lead content of water, in addition to the normal dietary intake, still assuming a 15 per cent uptake from the gut similar to food, the contribution of water of concentration 100 μg/l and volume drunk 1.25 l would be 19 μg/day to the absorption, giving a total increased absorption of 46 μg/day. If one assumes that the relationship between absorption and blood lead is linear, this would give a blood lead concentration of 26 μg/100 ml, corresponding to an increase of 8.8 μg%/100 μg/day. Experimental studies, however, show that the kind of increase likely to be expected from this increased exposure will be half this figure and the explanation ultimately lies in the non-linear relationship between intake and blood lead (Moore *et al.*, 1977, 1979; Sherlock *et al.*, 1982).

From all that has been said, it is clear that there are some discrepancies between these experimental calculations and the actual changes in blood lead with respect to change in both gastrointestinal and pulmonary exposure. There are only two possible explanations of this. First, that an important but unquantified source of exposure has not been included in the calculations. This would seem unlikely. Secondly, that the relationship between blood lead and lead intake is non-linear. This hypothesis is supported by both the non-linear relationship between water lead exposure and blood lead concentrations (DHSS, 1980) and by the habituation effect observed in rats and in sheep during long-term exposure to lead (Morrison *et al.*, 1974, Moore *et al.*, 1975).

This is very important in consideration of the probable contributions to blood lead and excreted lead from absorbed lead in industrial workers, since these subjects are exposed to very much greater concentrations of lead in their working environment than would ever be found in normal living circumstances. All of the figures therefore calculated here are underestimates of the true total exposure, but give a good estimate of the probable relationships between gastrointestinal and pulmonary exposure and absorption, and do not minimise the potential relationship between 'fall-out' of lead from air onto foodstuffs and their contributory significance to overall dietary exposure.

In conclusion, therefore, a compartmental model of the type demonstrated here which represents man as an environmental system, can be analysed through solution of time-dependent equations which describe transport of lead in the body, generally assuming first-order kinetics. Alternatively, the time-independent co-efficients between the different compartments can be determined to evaluate the exposure commitment and to relate these to steady-state concentrations in the various compartments of the pathway (O'Brien, 1979).

Overview

The human organism is thus seen to be one in which there is a considerable variation in the distribution of this metal. Concentrations range from values as low as $10^{-8}M$ in body fluids to as high as $10^{-4}M$ in bone (on a weight per weight basis) with soft tissue concentrations lying intermediate between these two values, but generally in the range $10^{-7} - 10^{-6}$M. Because of the proven toxic effects of this metal, it is therefore of some concern that such potentially high concentrations can be reached. There is for instance very little margin of safety in the normal level of lead present in blood, around $0.5 - 1 \times 10^{-6}$M when one realises that toxic effects of lead are found when blood levels rise to values of only 2×10^{-6}M. It has been argued that in prehistoric times man was exposed to much lesser quantities of lead in his general environment, and this was probably so, but whether or not this genuinely resulted in markedly lower levels of lead in the blood and tissues must be a matter of conjecture, since the relationship between exposure and levels in the blood appears to show a large rate of change at the lowest levels of exposure, according to proposed non-linear models. There is certainly greater storage of lead in bones at the present time, but such stored material does not ordinarily present a toxic hazard unless mobilised.

Of much more consequence, therefore, is that component of the metal which is free, unbound to any tissue, able to move freely to a site of action and there to cause its various deleterious effects. To this end there would appear to be some ability of the human organism to protect itself against this toxic insult. The non-linear relationship described earlier is one such mechanism. Others would be to increase excretory rates, or to increase the quantities of bound material, possibly through formation of specific binding proteins (Oskarsson *et al.*, 1982; Shelton and Egle, 1982). The most specific of these proteins described to date has been haemoglobin, and in particular the gamma globin of fetal haemoglobin. It is remarkable that this particular compound is, with its high oxygen affinity, seen to increase in lead poisoning and this certainly points to a reversal change in the haemoglobin 'switch' which could be interpreted as a protective mechanism to cover the relative metabolic anoxia induced by lead poisoning.

Lead, therefore, is present in considerable quantities in modern man's environment, and consequently, also in modern man. The toxic effects of the metal have resulted in moves to abate its environmental impact. It is unlikely that we will ever return to the halcyon pre-plumbous days of pre-industrial environmental exposure but abatement has already had encouraging and measurable effects on bodily levels of lead in the industrialised human.

References

Alessio, L., Castoldi, M.R., Monelli, O., Toffoletto, F. and Zochetti, C. (1979) Indicators of internal dose in current and past exposure to lead. *Int. Arch. Occup. Environ. Health, 44,* 127-32.

Alexander, F.W., Clayton, B.E. and Delves, H.T. (1974) Mineral and trace metal balances in children receiving normal and synthetic drugs. *Quart. J. Med., 43,* 89-111.

Al-Naimi, T., Edmonds, M.I. and Fremlin, J.H. (1980) The distribution of lead in human teeth, using charged particle activation analysis. *Phys. Med. Biol..,* 25, 719-26.

Anders, E., Bagnell, C.R., Krigman, M.R. and Mushak, P. (1982) Influence of dietary protein composition on lead absorption in rats. *Bull. Environ. Contam. Toxicol., 28,* 61-7.

Annest, J.L., Pirkle, J.L., Makuc, D., Neese, J.W., Bayse, D.D. and Kovar, M.G. (1983) Chronological trends in blood lead levels between 1976 and 1980. *N. Engl. J. Med., 308,* 1373-7.

Archer, A. and Barratt, T. (1976) Lead in the environment. *J. Roy. Soc. Health, 4,* 173-6.

Aufderheide, A.C., Neiman, F.D., Wittmers, L.E. and Rapp, G. (1981) Lead in bone. II Skeletal lead content as an indicator of lifetime lead ingestion and the social correlates in an Archaelogical population. *Am. J. Phys. Anthrop., 55,* 285-91.

Aungst, B.J., Dolce, J.A. and Fung, H.-L. (1981) The effect of dose on the disposition of lead in rats after intravenous and oral administration. *Toxicol. Appl. Pharmacol., 61,* 48-57.

—— and Fung, H.-L. (1981) Kinetic characterisation of in vitro lead transport across the rat small intestine. *Toxicol. Appl. Pharmacol., 61,* 39-47.

—— and —— Intestinal lead absorption in rats: effects of circadian rhythm, food, undernourishment, and drugs which alter gastric emptying and GI motility. *Res. Commun. Chem. Path. Pharmacol., 34,* 515-30.

Barltrop, D., Barrett, A.J. and Dingle, J.T. (1971) Subcellular distribution of lead in the rat. *J. Lab. Clin. Med., 77,* 705-12.

—— and Khoo, H.E. (1976) The influence of dietary minerals and fat on the absorption of lead. *Sci. Total Environ., 6,* 265-73.

—— and Meek F. (1979) Effect of particle size on lead absorption from the gut. *Arch. Environ. Health, 36,* 280-5.

—— and Smith, A. (1971) Interaction of lead with erythrocytes. *Experientia (Basel), 27,* 92-3.

Barry, P.S.I. (1975) A comparison of concentrations of lead in human tissues. *Br. J. Ind. Med., 32,* 119-39.

—— (1981) Concentrations of lead in the tissues of children. *Br. J. Ind. Med., 38,* 61-71.

—— (1981) Additional set of data in support of concentrations of lead in the tissue of children. *Br. J. Ind. Med., 38.*

—— and Connolly, R. (1981) Lead concentrations in mediaeval bones. *Int. Arch. Occup. Environ. Health, 48,* 173-7.

Barton, J.C. and Conrad, M.E. (1981) Effect of phosphate on the absorption and retention of lead in the rat. *Am. J. Clin. Nutr., 34,* 2192-8.

——, —— Harrison, L. and Nuby, S. (1978) Effects of calcium on the absorption and retention of lead. *J. Lab. Clin. Med., 92,* 366-76.

——, ——, —— and —— (1980) Effects of vitamin D on the absorption and retention of lead. *Am. J. Physiol., 238,* G124-G130.

——, —— and Holland, R. (1981) Iron, lead and cobalt absorption: similarities and dissimilarities. *Proc. Soc. Exp. Biol. Med., 166,* 64-9.

——, ——, Nuby, S. and Harrison, L. (1978) Effects of iron on the absorption and retention of lead. *J. Lab. Clin. Med.*, *92*, 536-47.

Batschelet, E., Brand, L. and Steiner, A. (1979) On the kinetics of lead in the human body. *J. Math. Biol.*, *8*, 15-23.

Bell, R.R. and Spicket, J.T. (1981) The influence of milk in the diet on the toxicity of orally ingested lead in rats. *Fd. Cosmet. Toxicol.*, *19*, 429-36.

Berlin, A., Amavis, R. and Langevin, M. (1977) Research on lead in drinking water in Europe (in relation to the possible uptake of lead by man). WHO Working Group on Health Hazards from Drinking Water, London.

Bernard, S.R. (1977) Dosimetric data and metabolic model for lead. *Health Physics.*, *32*, 44-6.

Bessis, M.C. and Jensen, W.N. (1965) Sideroblastic anaemia, mitochondria and erythroblastic iron. *Br. J. Haematol.*, *11*, 49-51.

Blair, J.A., Coleman, I.P.L. and Hilburn, M.E. (1979) The transport of the lead cation across the intestinal membrane. *J. Physiol.*, *286*, 343-50.

Blake, K.C.H. (1976) Absorption of ^{203}Pb from gastrointestinal tract of man. *Environ. Res.*, *11*, 1-4.

—— (1980) *Radioactive Lead Studies in the Human.* PhD Thesis, University of Cape Town.

Box, V., Cherry, N., Waldron, H.A., Dattani, J., Griffiths, K.D. and Hill, F.G.H. (1981) Plasma vitamin D and blood lead concentrations in Asian children. *Lancet, ii*, 373.

Brudevold, F., Aasenden, R., Srinivasian, B.N. and Bakhos, Y. (1977) Lead in enamel and saliva, dental caries and the use of enamel biopsies for measuring past exposure to lead. *J. Dent. Res.*, *56*, 1165-71.

—— and Steadman, L.T. (1956) The distribution of lead in human enamel. *J. Dent. Res.*, *35*, 430-7.

Bushnell, P.J. and DeLuca, H.F. (1981) Lactose facilitates the intestinal absorption of lead in weanling rats. *Science, 211*, 61-3.

—— and Levin, E.D. (1983) Effects of zinc deficiency on lead toxicity in rats. *Neurobehav. Toxicol. Teratol.*, *5*, 283-8.

Castellino, N. and Aloj, S. (1969) Intracellular distribution of lead in the liver and kidney of the rat. *Br. J. Ind. Med.*, *26*, 139-45.

Centre for Disease Control (1982) Blood lead levels in US population. *Morbidity and Mortality Weekly report*, *31*, 132-4.

Cerklewski, F.L. (1983) Influence of maternal magnesium deficiency on tissue lead content of rats. *J. Nutr.*, *113*, 1443-7.

—— and Forbes, R.M. (1976) Influence of dietary zinc on lead toxicity in the rat. *J. Nutr.*, *106*, 689-96.

Chamberlain, A.C., Heard, M.J., Little, P., Newton, D., Wells, A.C. and Wiffen, R.D. (1978) *Investigations into Lead from Motor Vehicles.* Environ. Med. Sci. Div., AERE, Harwell, HMSO, London.

——, ——, Stott, A.N.B., Clough, W.S., Newton, D. and Wells, A.C. (1975) Uptake of inhaled lead from motor exhaust. *Postgrad. Med. J.*, *51*, 790-4.

Clarkson, T.W. and Kench, J.E. (1958) Uptake of lead by human erythrocytes in vitro. *Biochem. J.*, *69*, 432-9.

Coleman, I.P.L., Hilburn, M.E. and Blair, J.A. (1978) The intestinal absorption of lead. *Biochem. Soc. Trans.*, pp. 915-17.

Conrad, M.E. and Barton, J.C. (1978) Factors affecting the absorption and excretion of lead in the rat. *Gastroenterology, 74*, 731-40.

Cooper, W.C. (1976) Cancer mortality patterns in the lead industry. *Ann. NY Acad. Sci.*, *271*, 250-9.

—— and Gaffey, W.R. (1975) Mortality of lead workers. *J. Occup. Med.*, *17*, 100-7.

Coulston, F., Goldberg, L., Griffin, T.B. and Russell, J.C. (1972) *The Effects of Continuous Exposure to Airborne Lead 1, 2, 4.* Report to the US EPA.

Day, A.G., Evans, G. and Robson, L.E. (1977) *An Environmental Impact Study of an Urban Motorway.* City of Bristol. Environmental Health Department.

De la Burdé, B. and Shapiro, I.M. (1975) Dental lead, blood lead and pica in urban children. *Arch. Environ. Health, 30,* 281-4.

Delves, H.T., Clayton, B.E., Carmichael, A., Bubear, M. and Smith, M. (1982) An appraisal of the analytical significance of tooth-lead measurements as possible indices of environmental exposure of children to lead. *Ann. Clin. Biochem., 19,* 329-37.

DHSS (1980) *Lead and Health.* Report of the Working Party on Lead in the Environment (The Lawthor Report), HMSO, London.

Dobbins, A., Johnson, D.R. and Nathan, P. (1978) Effect of exposure to lead on maturation of intestinal iron absorption of rats. *J. Toxicol. Environ. Health, 4,* 541-50.

Department of the Environment (DOE) (1978) *Lead Pollution in Birmingham.* DOE, Pollution Paper No. 13, HMSO. London.

—— (1982) *The Glasgow Duplicate Diet Study* (1979/80) DOE (1982), Pollution Report, No. 11, HMSO, London.

El-Gazzar, R.M., Finelli, V.N., Boiano, J. and Petering, H.G. (1978) Influence of dietary zinc on lead toxicity in rats. *Toxicol. Lett., 1,* 227-34.

Erickson, J.E., Shirahata, H, and Patterson, C.C. (1979) Skeletal concentrations of lead in ancient Peruvians. *N. Engl. J. Med., 300,* 946-51.

Facchetti, S., Geiss, F., Gaglione, P., Colombo, A., Garibaldi, G., Spallanzani, G. and Gilli, G. (1982) *Istopic Lead Experiment.* Commission of the European Communities, Luxembourg.

Fine, B.P., Barth, A., Sheffet, A. and Lavenhar, M.A. (1976) Influence of magnesium on the intestinal absorption of lead. *Environ. Res., 12,* 224-7.

Flanagan, P.R., Hamilton, D.L., Haist, J. and Valberg, L.S. (1979) Inter-relationships between iron and lead absorption in iron-deficient mice. *Gastroenterology, 77,* 1074-81.

Fosse, G., Berg, N.P. and Justesen, M.S. (1978) Lead in deciduous teeth of Norwegian children. *Arch. Environ. Health, 33,* 166-75.

Furia, T.E. (1968) *Handbook of Food Additives,* Chemical Rubber Publ. Co., Cleveland. pp. 263-6; 289-312.

Garber, B.T. and Wei, E. (1974) Influence of dietary factors on the gastrointestinal absorption of lead. *Toxicol. Appl. Pharmacol., 27,* 685-91.

Gerber, G.B. and Deroo, J. (1975) Absorption of radioactive lead (^{210}Pb) by different parts of the intestine in young and adult rats. *Environ. Physiol. Biochem., 5,* 314-18.

Goldberg, A., Smith, J.A. and Lochhead, A.C. (1963) Treatment of lead poisoning with oral penicillamine. *Br. Med. J., i,* 1270-50.

Goyer, R.A. (1978) Calcium and lead interactions: some new insights. *J. Lab. Clin. Med., 91,* 363-5.

Grandjean, P., Nielsen, O.V. and Shapiro, I.M. (1979) Lead retention in ancient nubian and contemporary populations. *J. Environ. Pathol. Toxicol., 2,* 781-7.

Gross, S.B. (1981) Human oral and inhalation exposures to lead: summary of Kehoe balance experiments. *J. Toxicol. Environ. Health, 8,* 333-7.

——, Peitzer, E.A., Yaeger, D.W. and Kehoe, R.A. (1975) Lead in human tissues. *Toxicol. Appl. Pharmacol., 32,* 638-51.

Grunden, N., Stantic, M. and Buben, M. (1974) Influence of lead on calcium strontium transfer through the duodenal wall in rats. *Environ. Res., 8,* 203-6.

Hamilton, D.L. (1978) Inter-relationships of lead and iron retention in iron deficient mice. *Toxicol. Appl. Pharmacol., 46,* 651-61.

Hammond, P.B., O'Flaherty, E.J. and Gartside, P.S. (1979) The impact of ambient air lead on uptake and retention of lead in man – A critique of the recent literature, in *Management and Control of Heavy Metals in the Environment*, CEP Consultants, Edinburgh, London, pp. 93-4.

Harrison, G.E., Carr, T.E.F., Sutton, A., Humphreys, E.R. and Rundo, J., (1969) Effect of alginate on the absorption of lead in man. *Nature, 224*, 1115-16.

Harrison, R.M. and Laxen, D.P.H. (1981) *Lead Pollution. Causes and Control.* Chapman and Hall, London.

Hart, M.H. and Smith, J.L. (1981) Effect of vitamin D and low dietary calcium on lead uptake and retention in rats. *J. Nutr., 4*, 694-8.

Heard, M.J. and Chamberlain, A.C. (1982) Effect of minerals and food on uptake of lead from the gastrointestinal tract in humans. *Human Toxicol., 1*, 411-15.

Hilburn, M.E., Coleman, I.P.L. and Blair, J.A. (1980) Factors influencing the transport of lead across the small intestine of the rat. *Environ. Res., 23*, 301-8.

Hohnadel, D.C., Sunderman, F. W., Nechay, M.W. and McNeely, M.D. (1973) Atomic absorption spectrometry of nickel, copper, zinc and lead in sweat collected from healthy subjects during sauna bathing. 1.2. *Clin. Chem., 19*, 1288-92.

Honigsmann, H., Jahn, O. and Bauer, E. (1974) Bleivergiftung; feinstrukturelle lokalisation von vlei im gingivagewebe. *Int. Arch. Arbeitsmed., 32*, 129-44.

Holtzman, R.B., Lucas, H.F. and Ilcewicz, F.H. (1968) *Concentration of Lead in Human Bone.* Argonne National Laboratory Publication No. ANL-7615, pp. 43-9.

Horiuchi, K., Horiguchi S. and Suekane, M. (1959) Studies on industrial lead poisoning. *Osaka City Med. J., 5*, 41-70.

Hursh, J.B. and Mercer, T.T. (1970) Measurement of ^{212}Pb loss rate from human lungs. *J. Appl. Physiol., 28*, 268-74.

—— and Suomela, J. (1968) Absorption of ^{212}Pb from the gastrointestinal tract of man. *Acta Radiol., 7*, 108-20.

IRCP (1975) *Task Group Report on a Reference Man.* International Commission on Radiological Protection, Publication 23, Pergammon Press, Oxford.

Joselow, M.M. and Bogden, J.D. (1977) Lead content of printed media (warning: spitballs may be hazardous to your health). *Am. J. Public Health, 64*, 238-40.

Jugo, J., Maljkovic, T. and Kostial, K, (1975) Influence of chelating agents on the gastrointestinal absorption of lead. *Toxicol. Appl. Pharmacol., 34*, 259-68.

Kaneko, Y., Inamori, I. and Nishimura, M. (1974) Zinc, lead, copper and cadmium in human teeth from different geographical areas in Japan. *Bull. Tokyo Dent. Coll, 15*, 233-43.

Kaplan, M.L., Jones, A.G., David, M.A. and Kopito, L. (1976) Inhibitory effect of iron on the uptake of lead by erythrocytes. *Life Sci., 16*, 1545-54.

Kehoe, R.A. (1961) The metabolism of lead in man in health and disease – Harben Lectures 1960 *J. Roy. Inst. Publ. Health Hyg., 24*, 1-203.

——, Cholak, J., Hubbard, D.N., Bambach, K., McNary, R.R. and Story, R.V. (1943) Experimental studies on ingestion of lead compounds. *J. Ind. Hyg., 25*, 71-9.

Keller, C.A. and Doherty, R.A. (1980) Effect of dose on lead retention and distribution in suckling and adult female mice. *Toxicol. Appl. Pharmacol., 52*, 285-93.

Kelliher, D.J., Hilliard, E.P., Poole, D.B.R. and Collins, J.D. (1973) The absorption of lead. *Irish J. Agric. Res., 12*, 61-9.

Klauder, D.S. and Petering, H.G. (1975) Protective value of dietary copper and iron against some toxic effects of lead in rats. *Environ. Health Perspect., 12*, 77-80.

Klevay, L.M. and Hyg, S.D. (1973) Hair as a biopsy material. III Assessment of environmental lead exposure. *Arch. Environ. Health, 26,* 169-72.

Kostial, K and Kello, D. (1979) Bioavailability of lead in rats fed 'human' diets. *Bull. Environ. Contam. Toxicol., 21,* 312-14.

——, Maljkovic, T. and Jugo, S. (1974) Lead acetate toxicity in rats in relation to age and sex. *Arch. Toxicol., 31,* 265-9.

Lacey, R.F., Moore, M.R. and Richards, W.N. (1985) Lead in water, infant diet and blood. The Glasgow Duplicate Diet Study. *Science of the Total Environment., 41,* 235-57.

Lawther, P.J., Commins, B.T., Ellison, J. McK. and Biles, B. (1973) More observations on airborne lead, in *Environmental Health Aspects of Lead.* Commission of the European Communities, Luxembourg, pp. 373-89.

Lockeretz, W. (1975) Lead content of deciduous teeth of children in different environments. *Arch. Environ. Health, 30,* 583-7.

Mackie, A.C., Stephens, R., Townshend, A. and Waldron, H.A. (1977) Tooth lead levels in Birmingham children. *Arch. Environ. Health, 32,* 178-85.

Mahaffey, K.R. (1980) Nutrient lead interactions, in R.L. Singhal and J.A. Thomas (eds). *Lead Toxicity.* Urban and Schwarzenberg, Baltimore and Munich, pp. 425-60.

——, Annest, J.L. Barbano, H.E. and Murphy, R.S. (1979) Preliminary analysis of blood lead concentrations for children and adults Nhanes II 1976-1980, in D.D. Hemphill (ed). *Trace Substances in Environmental Health, XIII.* University of Missouri, Columbia, pp. 37-57.

——, Goyer, R.A. and Wilson, M.H. (1974) The influence of ethanol ingestion on lead toxicity in rats fed isocaloric diets. *Arch. Environ. Health, 28,* 217-22.

Malik, S.R. and Fremlin, J.H. (1974) A study of lead distribution in human teeth, using charged particle activation analysis. *Caries Res., 8,* 283-92.

Marcus, A.H. (1979) The body burden of lead: comparison of mathematical models for accumulation. *Environ. Res., 19,* 79-90.

McNiff, E.F., Cheng, L.K., Woodfield, H.C. and Fung, H.L. (1978) Effects of L-cysteine, L-cysteine derivatives and ascorbic acid on lead excretion in rats. *Res. Commun. Chem. Pathol. Pharmacol., 20,* 131-7.

Meredith, P.A., Moore, M.R. and Goldberg, A. (1977) Effects of aluminium, lead and zinc on delta-aminolaevulinic acid dehydratase. *Enzyme, 22,* 22-7.

——, —— and —— The effect of calcium on lead absorption in rats. *Biochem. J., 166,* 531-7.

Moore, M.R. (1975) Lead and the mitochondrion. *Postgrad. Med. J., 51,* 760-4.

—— (1979) Diet and lead toxicity. *Proc. Nutr. Soc., 38,* 243-50.

—— (1980) Prenatal exposure to lead and mental retardation, in H.L. Needleman (ed.) *Health Effects of Lead at Low Dose.* Raven Press, NY, pp.53-65.

——, Campbell, B.C., Meredith, P.A., Beattie, A.D., Goldberg, A. and Campbell, D. (1978) The association between lead concentrations in teeth and domestic water lead concentrations. *Clin. Chim. Acta, 87,* 77-83.

—— and Goldberg, A. (1983) Health implications of the haemopoietic effects of lead, in K.R. Mahaffey (ed.) *Health Consequences of Current Levels of Environmental Lead Exposure.* Elsevier, Amsterdam.

——, Hughes, M.A. and Goldberg, D.J. (1979) Lead absorption in man from dietary sources. *Int. Arch. Occup. Environ. Health, 44,* 81-90.

——, McColl, K.E.L. and Goldberg, A. (1983) Porphyrins and alcohol, in Rosalki, S.B. (ed.) *Clinical Biochemistry of Alcoholism.* Churchill Livingstone.

——, Meredith, P.A., Campbell, B.C., Goldberg, A. and Baird, A.W. (1978) The effects of calcium glycerophosphate on industrial and experimental lead absorption. *Drugs Exp. Clin. Res., 4,* 17-24.

——, ——, ——, —— and Pocock, S.J. (1977) Contribution of lead in drinking water to blood lead. *Lancet, ii* 661-2.

——, ——, Goldberg, A., Carr, K.E., Toner, P.B., and Lawrie, T.D.V. (1975) Cardiac effects of lead in drinking water of rats. *Clin. Sci. Molec. Med., 49,* 337-41.

——, ——, Watson, W.S. and Campbell, B.C. (1979) The gastrointestinal absorption of 203 lead chloride in man, in D.D. Hemphill (ed). *13th Conference on Trace Substances in Environmental Health,* University of Missouri, Columbia, pp. 368-73.

Morrison, J.N., Quarterman, J. and Humphries, W.R. (1974) Lead metabolism in lambs and the effect of phosphate supplements. *Proc. Nutr. Soc., 33,* 88A.

Morrow, P.E., Beiter, H., Amato, F. and Gibb, F.R. (1980) Pulmonary retention of lead: an experimental study in man. *Environ. Res., 21,* 373-84.

Mouw, D.R., Wagner, J.G., Kalitis, K., Vander, A.J. and Mayor, G.H. (1978) The effect of parathyroid hormone on the renal accumulation of lead. *Environ. Res., 15,* 20-7.

Mykkänen, H. and Wasserman, R.H. (1981) Gastrointestinal absorption of lead (^{203}Pb) in chicks: influence of lead, calcium and age. *J. Nutr., 111,* 1757-65.

Mylius, E.A. and Ophus, E.M. (1977) Pulmonary distributions of lead in human subjects. *Bull. Environ. Contam. Toxicol., 17,* 302-10.

Mylroie, A.A., Moore, L., Olyai, B. and Anderson, M. (1978) Increased susceptibility to lead toxicity in rats fed semipurified diets. *Envon. Res., 15,* 57-64.

National Academy of Sciences (1980) *Lead in the Human Environment.* Washington DC.

Needleman, H.L., Davidson, I., Sewell, E.M. and Shapiro, I.M. (1974) Subclinical lead exposure in Philadelphia schoolchildren. Identification by denture lead analysis. *N. Engl. J. Med, 290,* 245-8.

——, Tuncay, O.C. and Shapiro, I.M. (1972) Lead levels in deciduous teeth of urban and suburban American children. *Nature, 235,* 111-12.

O'Brien, B.J. (1979) The exposure commitment method with application to exposure of man to lead pollution. MARC Technical Report, No. 13.

——, Smith, S. and Coleman, D.O., (1980) Lead Pollution of the Global Environment. Monitoring and Assessment Research Centre. Technical Report No. 16.

Ong, C.N. (1980) *Uptake and Interaction of Lead 203 with Human Peripheral Blood in vitro.* PhD Thesis, University of Liverpool.

—— and Lee, W.R. (1980) Interaction of calcium and lead in human erythrocytes. *Br. J. Ind. Med., 37,* 70-7.

—— and —— (1980) Distribution of lead 203 in human peripheral blood *in vitro. Br. J. Ind. Med., 37,* 78-84.

—— and —— (1980) High affinity of lead for fetal haemoglobin. *Br. J. Ind. Med., 37,* 292-8.

Oskarsson, A., Squibb, K.S. and Fowler, B.A. (1982) Intracellular binding of lead in the kidney: The partial isolation and characterisation of postmitochondrial lead binding components. *Biochem. Biophys. Res. Commun., 104,* 290-8.

Parmley, R.T., Barton, J.C., Conrad, M.E. and Austin, R.L. (1979) Ultrastructural radioautography and cytochemistry of lead absorption. *Am. J. Pathol., 96,* 85-100.

Peaslee, M.H. and Einhellig, F.A. (1977) Protective effect of tannic acid in mice receiving dietary lead. *Experientia, 33,* 1206.

Peng, T.-C., Gitelman, H.J. and Garner, S.C. (1979) Acute lead-introduced increase in serum calcium in the rat without increased secretion of calcitonin *Proc. Soc. Exp. Biol. Med., 160,* 114-17.

Pfrieme, F. (1934) Uber den normalen und pathologischen bleigeheld der Zahne von menschen und tieren. *Arch. Hyg., 111,* 232-43.

Pinchin, M.J., Newham, J. and Thompson, R.P.J. (1978) Lead, copper and cadmium in teeth of normal and mentally retarded children. *Clin. Chim. Acta, 85*, 89-94.

Plechaty, M.M., Noll, B. and Sunderman, F.W. (1977) Lead concentrations in semen of healthy men without occupational exposure to lead. *Ann. Clin. Lab. Sci., 7*, 515-18.

Quarterman, J., Humphries, W.R., Morrison, J.N. and Morrison, E. (1980) The influence of dietary amino acids on lead absorption. *Environ. Res., 23*, 54-67.

—— and Morrison, E. (1978) The effect of age on the absorption and excretion of lead. *Environ. Res., 17*, 78-83.

——, Morrison, E., Morrison, J.N. and Humphries, W.R. (1978) Dietary protein and lead retention. *Environ. Res., 17*, 68-77.

—— and Morrison, J.N. (1975) The effects of dietary calcium and phosphorus on the retention and excretion of lead in rats. *Br. J. Nutr., 34*, 351.

——, —— and Humphries, W.R. (1976) The effects of dietary lead content and food restriction on lead retention in rats. *Environ. Res., 12*, 180-7.

——, ——, —— and Mills, C.F. (1977) The effect of dietary sulphur and of castration on lead poisoning in lambs. *J. Comp. Pathol., 87*, 405-16.

Rabinowitz, M.B., Kopple, J.D. and Wetherill, G.W. (1980) Effect of food intake and fasting on gastrointestinal lead absorption in humans. *Am. J. Clin. Nutr., 33*, 1784-8.

—— and Needleman, H.L. (1982) Temporal trends in the lead concentrations of umbilical cord blood. *Science, 216*, 1429-31.

—— and —— (1983) Petrol lead sales and umbilical cord blood lead levels in Boston, Massachusetts. *Lancet, i*, 63.

——, Wetherill, G.W. and Kopple, J.D. (1973) Lead metabolism in the normal human: stable isotope studies. *Science, 182*, 725.

——, —— and —— (1976) Kinetic analysis of lead metabolism in healthy humans. *J. Clin. Invest., 58*, 260-70.

Ragan, H.E. (1977) Effects of iron deficiency on the absorption and distribution of lead and cadmuim in rats. *J. Lab. Clin. Med., 90*, 700-6.

Rao, D.V. and Goodwin, P.N. (1973) 203 Pb: a potential radionuclide for skeletal imaging. *J. Nucl. Med., 14*, 872.

Rastogi, S.C., Clausen, J. and Srivastava K.C. (1976) Selenium and lead: mutual detoxifying effects. *Toxicology, 6*, 377-88.

Renshaw, G.D., Pounds, C.A. and Pearson, E.F. (1972) Variation in lead concentration along single hairs as measured by non-flame atomic absorption spectrophotometry. *Nature, 238*, 162.

Robertson, I.K. and Worwood, M. (1978) Lead and iron absorption from rat small intestine: the effect of dietary Fe deficiency. *Br. J. Nutr., 40*, 253-60.

Rosen, J.F., Chesney, R.W., Hamstra, A., Hector, M.S., DeLuca, F. and Mahaffey, K. (1980) Reduction in 1,25-dihydroxyvitamin D in children with increased lead absorption. *N. Engl. J. Med., 302*, 1128-31.

——, Zarate-Salvador, C. and Trinidad, E.E. (1974) Plasma lead levels in normal and lead intoxicated children. *J. Paediatr., 84*, 45-8.

Rytoma, I. and Tuompo, H. (1974) Lead levels in deciduous teeth. *Naturwissenschaften, 61*, 8.

Schroeder, H.A. and Tipton, I.H. (1968) The human body burden of lead. *Arch. Environ. Health, 17*, 965-78.

Schubert, J. and Lindenbaum, A. (1960) The mechanism of action of chelating agents on metallic elements in the intact animal. in J.J. Seven and L.A. Johnson (eds) *Metal Binding in Medicine*. Lippincott, Philadelphia. p.68.

Shah, B.G., Momcilovic, B. and McLaughlin, J.M. (1980) Increased retention of lead in young rats fed suboptimal protein and minerals. *Nutr. Rept. Int., 21*, 1-9.

Shapiro, I.M., Dobkin, B.T., Tuncay, O.C. and Needleman, H.L. (1973) Lead levels in dentine and circumpulpal dentine of deciduous teeth of normal and lead poisoned children. *Clin. Chim. Acta, 46,* 119-23.

——, Grandjean, P. and Nielson, O.V. (1980) Lead levels in bones and teeth of children in ancient Nubia: evidence of both minimal lead exposure and lead poisoning, in H.L. Needleman (ed.) *Low Level Lead Exposure.* Raven Press, New York, pp.35-42.

——, Mitchell, G., Davidson I. and Katz, S.H. (1975) The lead content of teeth. *Arch. Environ. Health, 30,* 483-90.

Shelton, K.R. and Egle, P.M. (1982) The proteins of lead induced nuclear inclusion bodies. *J. Biol. Chem., 257,* 11802-7.

Sherlock, J., Smart, G., Forbes, G.I., Moore, M.R., Patterson, W.J., Richards, W.N. and Wilson, T.S. (1982) Assessment of lead intakes and dose-response for a population in Ayr exposed to a plumbosolvent water supply. *Human Toxicol., 1,* 115-22.

Sinn, W. (1980) Uber den Zusammenhang von Luftbleikonzentraten und bleigehalt des blutes von Autohnern und Betrupstätngen in Kerngebeit einer Grosstadt. I *Int. Arch. Occup. Environ. Health, 47,* 93-118.

—— (1981) II. *Int. Arch. Occup. Environ. Health, 48,* 1-22.

Six, K.M. and Goyer, R.A. (1972) The influence of iron deficiency on tissue content and toxicity of ingested lead in the rat. *J. Lab. Clin. Med., 79,* 128-36.

Sleet, R.B. and Soares, J.H. (1978) Effects of vitamin E deficiency on tissue lead deposition and on hepatic xanthine dehydrogenase activity in the mallard duck. *Proc. West. Pharmacol. Soc., 21,* 481-2.

Smart, G.A., Warrington, M. and Evans, W.H. (1981) The contibution of lead in water to dietary lead intakes. *J. Sci. Fd. Agric., 32,* 129-33.

Smith, D., De Luca, H.F., Tanaka, Y. and Mahaffey, K.R. (1978) Stimulation of lead absorption by vitamin D administration. *J. Nutr., 108,* 843-7.

Snowdon, C.T. (1977) A nutritional basis for lead pica. *Phys. Behav., 18,* 885-93.

Sobel, A.E. and Burges, M. (1955) *J. Biol. Chem., 212,* 105-10.

Sorrell, M., Rosen, J.F. and Roginsky, M. (1977) Interactions of lead, calcium, vitamin D and nutrition in lead burdened children. *Arch. Environ. Health, 31,* 160-4.

Stack, M.V., Burkitt, A.J. and Nickless, G. (1975) Lead in children's teeth. *Nature, 255,* 169.

——, —— and —— (1976) Trace metals in teeth at birth (1957-1963 and 1972-1973) *Bull. Environ. Contam. Toxicol., 16,* 764-6.

Steadman, L.T., Brudevold, F., Smith, F.A., Gardner, D.E. and Little, M.F. (1959) Trace elements in ancient Indian teeth. *J. Dent. Res., 38,* 285-91.

Steenhout, A. and Pourtois, M. (1981) Lead accumulation in teeth as a function of age with different exposures. *Br. J. Ind. Med., 38,* 297-303.

Stephens, R. and Waldron, H.A. (1975) The influence of milk and related dietary constituents on lead metabolism. *Fd. Cosmet. Toxicol., 13,* 555-63.

Stewart, D.J. (1974) Teeth as indicators of exposure of children to lead. *Arch. Dis. Child., 49,* 895-7.

Strehlow, C.D. (1972) *The Use of Deciduous Teeth as Indicators of Lead Exposure.* PhD Thesis, New York University.

Suzuki, T. and Yoshida, A. (1979) Effect of dietary supplementation of iron and ascorbic acid on lead toxicity in rats. *J. Nutr., 109,* 982-8.

—— and —— (1979) Effectiveness of dietary iron and ascorbic acid in the prevention and cure of moderately long-term lead toxicity in rats. *J. Nutr., 109,* 1974-8.

Thawley, D.G., Willoughby, R.A., McSherry, B.J., MacLeod, G.K., MacKay K.H. and Mitchell, W.R. (1977) Toxic interactions among Pb, Zn and Cd with

varying levels of dietary Ca and vitamin D: haematological system. *Environ. Res., 14*, 463-75.
Tokarski, E. and Reio, L. (1978) Effect of lead poisioning on the thiamine status and function in liver and blood of rats. *Acta Chem. Scand., B32*, 375-9.
Tsuchiya, K., Sugita, A., Seki, Y., Kobayashi, Y., Hori, M. and Park, C.B. (1975) Study of lead concentrations in atmosphere and population in Japan, in T.B. Griffin and J.H. Knelson (eds) *Lead.* Academic Press, London.
Vostal, J. (1966) Study of the renal excretory mechanisms of heavy metals. *15th International Conference on Occupational Health, Vienna*, pp. 61-4.
Waldron, H.A (1982) Lead in bones: a cautionary tale. *Ecol. Dis., 1*, 191-6.
—— and Stofen, D. (1974) *Subclinical Lead Poisoning.* Academic Press, London, New York.
Watson, W.S., Hume, R. and Moore, M.R. (1980) Oral absorption of lead and iron. *Lancet, ii*, 236-7.
Wilkinson, D.R. and Palmer, W. (1975) Lead in teeth as a function of age. *Am. Lab., 41*, 67-70.
Wise, A. (1981) Protective action of calcium phytate against acute lead toxicity in mice. *Bull. Environ. Contam. Toxicol., 27*, 630-3.
WHO (1977) *Environmental Health Criteria 3, Lead.* World Health Organization, Geneva.
Ziegler, E.E., Edwards, B.B., Jensen, R.L., Mahaffey, K.R. and Fomon, S.J. (1978) Absorption and retention of lead by infants. *Pediat. Res., 12*, 29-34.
Zielhuis, R.L., (1975) Dose response relationships for inorganic lead. *Int. Arch. Occup. Environ. Health, 35*, 1-18.

6 THE DISTRIBUTION OF LEAD

Janet Hunter

Introduction

Lead reaches man from a variety of primary and secondary sources. These multiple pathways of intake, combined with the metabolic and social factors which influence exposure to lead and its rate of uptake into the body, are reflected in a non-random distribution of body lead levels in the human population. Excluding those occupationally exposed to lead, and their families, there is a risk of unduly high lead levels for people living in areas with plumbosolvent water, in inner cities where air and dust lead is high and near busy roads or local industrial lead sources. The risk is greatest in young, pre-school children.

Population Surveys

Much of the information in this chapter is derived from two recently completed large-scale surveys of population blood lead levels — one in the United Kingdom and one in the United States of America. The use of lead concentration in venous blood as the index of body lead burden is preferred in surveys of this size since it is relatively cheap and easy to assess over the whole population, quality control and therefore analytical precision is now well-established and blood lead concentration is a good indicator of current exposure to environmental lead.

The UK Screening Campaign for Lead

The UK screening campaign for lead (Pollution reports nos: 10 and 18, Quinn, 1983) was mounted in response to a European Community Directive requiring member states to carry out two blood lead screening campaigns separated by at least two years. The scheme was specifically aimed at adults in inner and outer urban areas and groups exposed to a significant source of lead pollution, excluding those exposed to lead in their jobs. The groups studied are therefore not a representative sample of the UK population and the results of the screening programme should not necessarily be generalised to lower risk groups.

The two UK EEC surveys took place during 1979 and 1981. In 1979 39 autonomous local surveys were carried out, consisting of 1800 randomly selected adults in the inner and outer urban areas of six major cities: 2000 children exposed to leadworks (either children of lead workers or children living near one of nine lead works), 300 adults and 500 children living near major roads, and 400 people exposed to high levels of lead in drinking water: 5000 people in total.

The 35 1981 surveys included 3500 people in all. Most of the surveys of children exposed to lead works were repeated while the emphasis for adults was on those with undue exposure to lead through living in older dwellings or near major roads. Most of the blood samples (over 95 per cent) were venous and blood lead was assessed by atomic absorption spectrometry according to stringent quality control criteria.

The blood lead results obtained were assessed in terms of 'reference levels' established by the EEC at the time the Directive was formulated: no more than 50 per cent of any group should have blood lead concentrations above 20 µg/100 ml, no more than 10 per cent should be above 30 µg/100 ml, and no more than 2 per cent should be above 35 µg/100 ml. Follow-up investigations were carried out in the UK for anyone with a blood lead concentration greater than 35 µg/100 ml and for any child over 30 µg/100 ml. Overall there were few breaches of the reference levels, these being in four groups exposed 'to high levels of lead in drinking water, three groups of children exposed to lead works where insufficient care was taken to control dust 'carry out', and one inner city sample living in older housing close to a busy road'.

Background information on each participant was collected by questionnaire.

The Second National Health and Nutrition Examination Survey (NHANES II)

The NHANES II survey (Annest *et al.*, 1983, Annest, 1983) was carried out in the USA from February 1976 to February 1980. A component of the survey was developed to measure the degree of exposure of the US population to certain toxic substances including lead. The overall sample of 27 801 people was selected according to a multistage probability design from the civilian, non-institutionalised population of the USA between 6 months and 74 years of age. The sample design provided for oversampling among those persons aged 6 months to 5 years, 60-74 years and those living in poverty areas. Of this sample 60.7 per cent (or 10049 people) gave blood specimens for blood lead determination. Nearly all (9933) were venous blood samples, the rest being capillary blood obtained by finger-prick. The blood lead assessments were made by atomic absorption spectrometry and the mean of duplicate analyses taken as the measure of blood lead concentration. Quality control methods were rigorous and included analysis of standard samples alongside every batch of experimental blood for the detection of time trends.

Social and medical data were also obtained from participants. The overall aim of the survey was to provide information about the distribution of blood lead levels in the US population, to establish base-line estimates for future studies of changes in exposure to lead over time, to provide normative data for use in health policy and to correlate lead levels with other health and nutritional parameters in the population under study. Children with blood lead concentrations of 30 μg/100 ml or more were referred for medical attention and follow-up tests in accordance with Center for Disease Control guidelines.

It must be emphasised when comparing the UK and US surveys that whereas the NHANES II blood lead data were collected from a representative sample of the US population, the UK EEC sample was aimed at particular target groups with expected high lead exposure and as such is not generalisable to the UK population as a whole.

In addition to these two major surveys several smaller scale blood lead studies of defined populations have been published, for example those carried out in Wales by the MRC Epidemiology Unit (Elwood, 1983) which are valuable in providing independent corroboration of the results of the large-scale work.

Distribution of Blood Lead Concentrations

Blood lead levels are distributed approximately log normally in the population as a whole and in most subgroups (Royal Commission 1983) that is, the majority of blood lead concentrations cluster around a mean value with a much smaller tail of higher leads (See

Figure 6.1: Frequency Distribution of Blood Lead Concentration in Adults Living in an Inner City Area (Manchester) and a Small Town (Llanybydder)

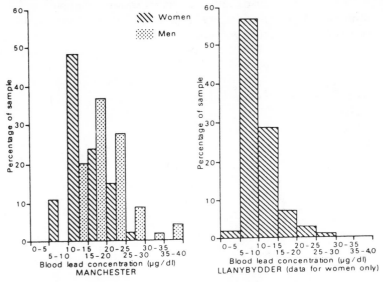

Source: Royal Commission on Environmental Pollution (1983), p. 49

Figure 6.1). This sort of distribution is to be expected for variables which have a fixed lower limit and an open upper end. However the mean values, and therefore the position of the distribution on the baseline may vary in association with various factors.

Although it is rare for one factor in isolation to be directly responsible for high blood lead levels, it is nevertheless possible to identify certain population subgroups as being at particular risk. In the sections that follow several contributory factors are considered.

Geographic Variation in Blood Lead Distribution

International Comparisons

The only recent world-wide blood lead screening programme of any size was that carried out by the World Health Organization (WHO) during 1980-81. The target populations were randomly selected groups of about 200 teachers from one urban area in each of ten countries from whom blood samples were taken for the

Figure 6.2: Concentrations of Lead in Blood (Median Values) for Male (M) and Female (F) Teachers, Subdivided into Smokers and Non-smokers (Including Former Smokers). Indian data represent teachers in Ahmedabad. Swedish data represent a random sample of the total population in Stockholm (1) Only 2 female smokers; (2) no female smokers

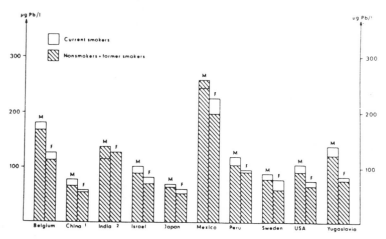

Source: Vahter (1982), p. 4

assessment of lead and cadmium levels according to strict quality control procedures. The UK did not participate.

Median blood lead concentrations were reported for males and females separately, subdivided into smokers and non-smokers (Vahter, 1982) for each participating country. The spread in blood lead levels among the countries was considerable — ranging from 6 µg/100 ml in China and Japan, to 22 µg/ 100 ml in Mexico. The WHO report on the surveys (Vahter, 1982) notes a relationship between blood lead values and exposure to lead in petrol: Mexico with the highest median blood lead levels also has the highest concentration of lead in petrol among the participating countries, in addition, Mexico City has very heavy vehicle traffic. In contrast, Tokyo, with one of the lowest median blood lead levels, despite being a large city with heavy traffic uses almost all unleaded fuel. However, other factors were undoubtedly involved since it was not possible to explain, for example, the relatively high blood lead levels found in some of the Indian cities by exposure to lead in petrol (See Figure 6.2).

Figure 6.3: European Community Blood Lead Survey, 1979: Median Blood Level Concentration in Adults and Children. Exposed/not exposed refers to the presence or absence of local industrial emissions of lead

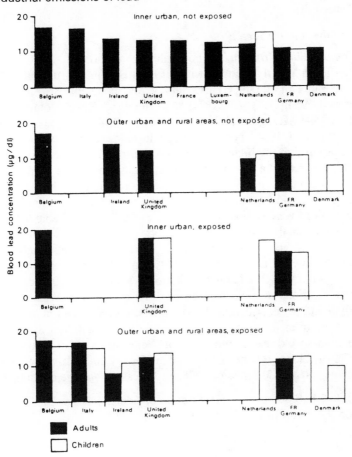

Source: Royal Commission on Environmental Pollution (1983)

The other recent international blood lead screening campaign is that carried out within the European community. It is possible to compare the results of the first EEC survey for the UK for adults from inner city communities not exposed to local industrial lead sources, with those of other member states (Royal Commission Report 1983). The United Kingdom blood lead values lie toward the centre of the range (mean 10.6 μg/100 ml) with those for Denmark and the Federal Republic of Germany being lowest and those of Belgium and Italy highest. The range of values found is, however, much smaller than that found in the WHO surveys (See Figure 6.3).

Within-Country Trends

Trends Within Britain.   Geographical variation in mean blood lead levels of urban adults within Great Britain was indicated by the results of the first EEC survey for six major British cities carried out in 1979 (DOE, 1981). The 1983 Royal Commission shows that average adult blood lead concentrations were lowest in London and 40-45 per cent higher in cities to the north. It was suggested that the higher average concentrations in the north may reflect increased exposure to environmental lead rather than social factors such as diet, in which case more plumbosolvent water supplies would be the most likely lead source since air lead concentrations were similar for all six cities studied (See Table 6.1).

Other smaller-scale studies report great area differences in blood lead concentrations, though differences in analytical methods mean that comparisons between, rather than within studies should be made with caution. Surveys of blood lead concentrations in adult women in different areas of Wales, both urban and rural, (Elwood, 1983) show a current mean blood lead concentration of about 11 μg/100 ml. Young children aged 1-3 years in an old lead mining area of Wales had a mean blood lead level of 23 μg/100 ml, compared to 18 μg/100 ml in a control village, (Royal Commission, 1983) whereas school-age children up

Table 6.1: Blood Lead Concentration of Adults in Major UK Cities from First European Community Survey, 1979

	Inner city μg/dl	Outer city μg/dl	Difference μg/dl
Birmingham	13.6	11.1	2.5
Greater London	12.0	10.2	1.8
Leeds	15.6	13.3	2.3
Liverpool	14.2	13.8	0.4
Manchester	17.0	16.6	0.4
Sheffield	14.6	13.2	1.4
All cities	12.8	11.0	1.8

Note: Figures are geometric means.
Source: Royal Commission on Environmental Pollution (1983), p. 49

to 8 years old in County Wicklow (Richardson, 1982) had a mean blood lead concentration of 7.1 µg/100 ml compared to children attending school in Dublin with a mean concentration of 16 µg/100 ml. Finally, pre-school children attending day-centres and nurseries in Birmingham (DOE, 1982) had a mean blood lead level of 20 µg/100 ml.

Most remarkable is a study of the population of a small, relatively inaccessible island lying 8 miles off the north-west coast of Ireland, using no petrol and having no piped water system (Elwood and Blaney, 1983). Mean blood lead concentrations for adult men were 8.9 µg/100 ml and 7.0 µg/100 ml for women — appreciably higher than might have been expected in comparison to the EEC findings for urban dwellers. Elwood and Blaney conclude that the most likely source for this lead is the diet of the islanders, due to an increased consumption of tinned food in recent years.

It is clear that these regional variations in blood lead concentrations in the UK cannot be explained by population density or industrial activity alone but are due to a complex of interacting local environmental and social factors.

Urban-Rural Differences.   A finding across different studies is that average blood lead levels in inner urban areas are consistently higher than in outer areas of the same cities and that blood lead concentrations of those living in rural areas are lower still.

The UK EEC studies were aimed at high risk groups and as such carried out no measures in rural populations not exposed to specific lead sources. The absolute mean levels of blood lead found in urban areas depended, as mentioned above, on geographical location, (Table 6.1) some northern outer city samples having higher mean blood lead concentrations than inhabitants of inner London. The consistent inner-outer zone differences found within the same city were in many cases attributable to a predominance of older housing (with the accompanying higher risk of lead exposure) in the inner city zones. After correcting for this, however, an average difference of about 1 µg/100 ml remained which, as Quinn (1983) suggests, corresponds closely with the expected effect due to differences in air lead concentrations.

The mean lead levels found in rural inhabitants by other British studies mentioned earlier suggest that rural dwellers may not have blood lead levels as low as those expected by extrapolation from

Figure 6.4: Mean Blood Lead Levels (PbB) of Children Ages 6 Months to 5 Years by Degree of Urbanisation: United States 1976-80

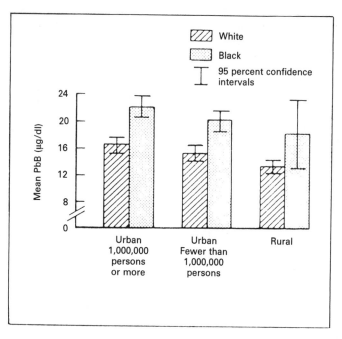

Source: Annest *et al.* (1982)

the inner/outer city comparisons. Indeed an investigation of two rural communities in south-west England, (Barltrop and Strehlow, 1982) found average blood lead levels of 9-10 μg/100 ml in both children and adults, very close to the mean level for outer London adults of 10.2 μg/100 ml.

The NHANES II results showed that urban dwellers had higher blood leads than rural dwellers. The difference was most pronounced in pre-school-aged children — 6 months to 5 years old (See Figure 6.4). The percentage of children with blood lead levels over the Center for Disease Control cut-off point for undue absorption (30 μg/100 ml) was also higher in inner city groups, particularly for black children.

It is likely for both the US and the UK that exposure to lead in inner city children is strongly influenced by socioeconomic factors such as income, diet, housing-type and available play space as well as environmental factors like the higher air lead levels due to higher traffic flow and proximity of industrial premises specifically associated with urban areas. In the US for example, the majority of black people sampled lived in urban areas and a large proportion of these had low incomes. The problem of the interactions between dwelling-place, race and income is discussed below.

Local Environmental Influences on Blood Lead Distribution

Age of Housing

In the UK EEC surveys it was found that blood lead concentrations in both adults and children living in homes built before 1945 were consistently higher (by a mean 1.5 μg/100 ml) than in those living in more modern accommodation. This is not surprising in that older houses are much more likely to have lead pipes in the domestic water system and to contain old paint with a high lead content. They may also harbour accumulated lead in dust from coal burning or, where there are local industrial sources, from past emissions. As mentioned above, age of housing is an important factor in accounting for inner versus outer city differences in blood lead levels.

There was no explicit measurement of blood lead by house age in the NHANES II study, but since older houses are more commonly found in poorer US inner city areas, house age may be an underlying factor accounting for some part of the consistent racial differences found within particular population subgroups, as explained below in the section on racial trends.

However, Hammond *et al.* (1983) reported a strong association between housing type and serial blood leads of high risk, urban children of 15-18 months in the US. The housing categories ranged from pre-World War II in deteriorated condition, to post-war public housing and paint was probably the main lead source.

Drinking Water

Exposure to soft, highly plumbosolvent domestic water supplies in Scotland was associated with the highest mean blood lead levels found during the UK EEC surveys in the most vulnerable groups of the population. Mean levels in mothers of young children in Ayr were 21 μg/100 ml whereas those for mothers and their children in Glasgow were 19.8 μg/100 ml and 20.8 μg/100 ml respectively.

Those living in pre-1945 houses had very much higher blood and water lead concentrations than those in post-1945 houses, indicating that much of the lead was derived from domestic plumbing. Though the Glasgow sample included deliberate oversampling of households with high lead levels in the domestic water supply the results gave rise to considerable concern. Following treatment of the water supplies by adding lime to increase alkalinity, there have been substantial falls in blood lead levels — in Glasgow around 20 per cent for adults and 25 per cent for bottle-fed infants.

Exposure to Lead Works

In the 1979 UK European Community Surveys, blood lead levels of children of lead workers and in those living around lead works were found to be elevated — a number having blood lead concentrations of over 30 µg/100 ml. As in other studies, e.g. Roels *et al.* (1980), blood lead levels in general decreased with increasing distance from the works. Since contamination from a lead works is mostly through increased dust lead as a result of fallout and carry-out by vehicles and workers, children are particularly vulnerable to this lead source. Measures taken to reduce emissions and to improve workers' hygiene following the 1979 surveys have had a substantial effect with reductions in blood lead in 1981 averaging about 20 per cent (over 3 µg/100 ml).

Major Roads

The UK EEC surveys found that mean blood lead levels of adults living near major roads were not very different from those in the general population in the same area — the same being true for children. Levels did decline slightly with increasing distance from a main road, but the effect was much less strong than that found for children living near lead works.

Demographic Influences on Blood Lead Distribution

Age, sex, socioeconomic status and race act indirectly to mediate the individual's exposure to lead sources and to affect the uptake of lead. They interact considerably in their effect and their combined influence identifies certain groups as being at particular risk for high lead levels.

Age

Concern about the more serious consequences of elevated body lead burden for the developing nervous system, together with the greater exposure of the young child to lead in dust (Roels *et al.*, 1980; Duggan, 1983; Royal Commission Report, 1983) means that age trends in blood lead level have been most closely studied for children, from birth to adolescence, particularly those at a high risk lead exposure. Though most studies are cross-sectional in design, their results agree surprisingly well, despite often being based on samples of very different populations.

The UK EEC surveys of an at-risk sample showed that mean blood lead increased steeply over the first two or three years of life

Figure 6.5: Blood Lead Concentration by Age of UK Children in the European Community Blood Lead Survey, 1979

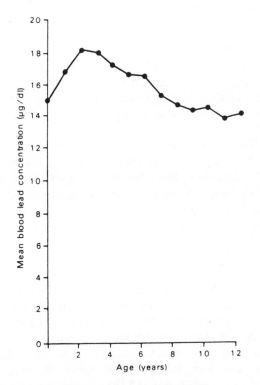

Figure 6.6: Blood Lead Levels in the United States

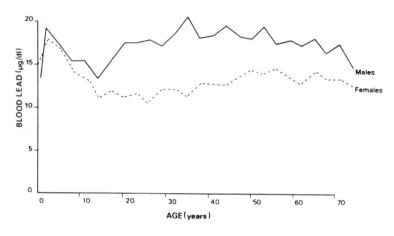

Source: Mahaffey *et al.,* (1979)

to a peak between 2 and 4 years, then began to decrease to a minimum at about the age of 12 years (Royal Commission Report 1983). Blood lead levels tended to remain fairly steady in adults, with a slight upward trend in males and a somewhat stronger trend in females. Levels in both sexes appear to stabilise during the mid-50s (See Figure 6.6).

The NHANES II survey found a similar trend in their random sample of the US population. There was a peak in early childhood followed by decreasing blood lead levels to about age 15 years in whites and to about 17 years in black children. Blood lead levels then increased steeply during adolescence, especially in men, levelling out to a gradual increase with age to around 45-54 years when they again began to decline (See Figure 6.6).

Hammond *et al.* (1983) reported on the blood lead profiles of children aged 0-2 years. By contrast with the above cross-sectional studies this is a longitudinal study and serial blood samples are taken from each child by venipuncture at three monthly intervals, beginning at birth with a cord blood sample. Though the families live in a deprived inner city area with a high incidence of elevated blood leads, the mean blood lead concentrations of the mothers, assessed around four months before the birth, were quite low (mean around 7 μg/100 ml). All the children were born with low

Figure 6.7: Blood Lead Profiles of Inner City Children Determined at three-month Intervals From Birth. The two profiles for individual children are the extremes for the study population. Numbers of subjects at each time point are indicated in parentheses. NHANES II data are for the US population known not to have unusual lead exposure

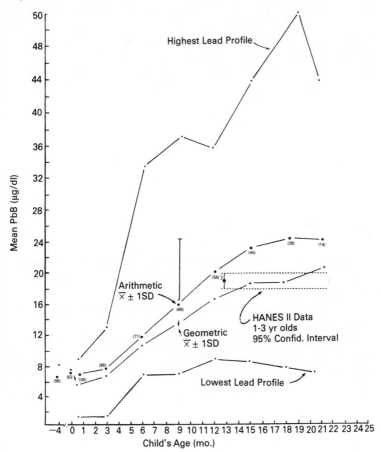

Source: Hammond *et al.* (1983), p. 265

cord blood lead levels — similar to those of their mothers — but their blood lead concentrations rose sharply between three and six months of age then diverged greatly, with peak blood lead levels so far ranging from 8 to 50 µg/100 ml (Figure 6.7). From six months onwards blood lead levels are highly predictive of subsequent blood lead levels.

The authors treated as surprising the sharp increase in blood lead level observed for virtually all the children between three and six months. Though no information on diet was presented, this may well coincide with the end of breast feeding and therefore with an increased intake of more lead-contaminated foods by the children. The steady, but less marked increase observed after six months was found to be strongly associated with the authors' definition of housing type — older housing in deteriorated condition being associated with higher blood lead levels. At 15-18 months, housing category accounted for 50 per cent of the variability in blood lead levels.

These results add support to the suggestion (Duggan, 1983) that dust lead is an important source of lead for young children. Children who are crawling rather than walking, and who continually mouth objects are highly exposed to lead in dust. Duggan also cites evidence that the early childhood peak in blood leads is small or absent altogether in children without much access to the general environment, such as hospitalised and institutionalised groups.

Sex

The influences of sex and age on population blood lead levels are strongly interactive. In general, sex differences in blood lead concentration seem to be negligible in younger children and to increase with age. For adults, men tend to have significantly higher blood leads than women.

The findings of two major UK surveys and the NHANES II survey with respect to sex differences are in close agreement despite the different populations under study. The UK EEC study found only very small differences between blood lead concentrations in lead exposed boys and girls up to age 12 but the adult males studied had average blood lead levels 30-35 per cent higher than those of the females. However, due to a stronger upward trend with age in women, the sex difference tended to decrease slightly in the mid-fifties and beyond.

An earlier population survey in Birmingham, UK (Department of the Environment, 1978) found a similar relationship between blood lead and sex, and showed that in this sample the male-female difference arose during adolescence (12-18 years) when the blood lead levels of the males but not the females, rose sharply

Figure 6.8: Blood Levels in Birmingham UK

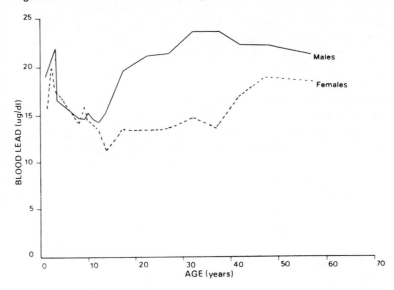

Source: Rutter and Jones (1983), p. 116

(See Figure 6.8).

The NHANES II results in turn showed that though young boys 6 months — 5 years old had slightly higher mean blood lead levels than girls of the same age, the differences were not statistically significant. In the 6-17 year age group the differences in blood lead levels increased more steeply for males until, for adults aged 18-74 years there was a pronounced and significant sex difference (cf. Figure 6.6). For adults, the mean blood lead levels of men are consistently higher than those of women in all age groups, though as observed in the UK samples, the steeper increase in blood lead with age in women means that the size of the mean difference decreases from about 6 μg/100 ml at age 35-44 years to around 4 μg/100 ml from 55 years onwards.

Additional evidence of a consistent male-female difference in blood lead concentrations is derived from the WHO cross-cultural survey (Vahter, 1982) where blood leads for adult males were on average 1.3 times higher than those for females.

Although the fact that significant sex differences in blood lead level do not appear until adolescence coupled with the known higher numbers of red blood cells and haemoglobin levels of men, seems to indicate some physiological basis for the sex difference in blood lead, it should be remembered that lead exposure in men and women is also very different. Men are likely to be more exposed to lead through their occupations, hobbies, DIY repair work, and through their greater smoking and drinking.

Socioeconomic Status

Socioeconomic status is typical of a factor which is used as a shorthand indicator of a great variety of other variables such as income, housing type, diet, education, attitude etc. As such, a unitary measure is bound to represent an oversimplifaction of the facts, so the problem when designing a study, is how to choose an appropriate measure which will be comparable across different populations.

The 1981 UK EEC surveys included questions on occupation and used the Registrar-General's Classification of Occupations (1980) to produce an index of 'social class' by ordering occupations into six major categories ranging from professional to unskilled manual. Children were classified according to the occupation of the head of the household. A problem with the Registrar-General's classification is that as an artificially constructed scale it is not metric, i.e. the difference between class I and II is not equal to the difference between class IV and V. Neither are the occupational categories equally represented in the population — classes I, IV and V are relatively under-represented while the majority of occupations fall into classes III manual and non-manual.

No clear, consistent differences in blood lead concentrations among the social classes were found for UK adults in the samples, but for children exposed to lead works, those whose parents were manual workers had blood lead levels on average 1 μg/100 ml higher than those of children of non-manual workers.

The NHANES II study used family income as its measure of socioeconomic status and found overall lower mean blood lead levels among the more affluent than among the poor (Figure 6.9). The three income categories used ranged from near the poverty threshold ($\leq$ $6000 p.a.), through $6000-14 000 p.a. to $15 000 and above. These income-related differences in blood lead were, however, most pronounced and statistically significant in children aged 6 months to 5 years.

A recent study carried out in the UK using tooth lead level as the index of body lead burden in a sample of urban children

Figure 6.9: Mean Blood Lead Levels (PbB) of Children Ages 6 Months–5 Years by Annual Family Income: United States, 1976-80

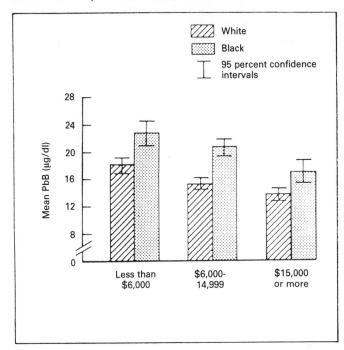

Source: Annest *et al.* (1982)

(Smith *et al.*, 1983) used a complex structured interview to identify specific items of the child's social, physical and emotional environment which might be related to lead uptake. Use of stepwise regressions to work out the interrelationships of those items most highly correlated with tooth lead found that a scale measuring family cleanliness accounted for the greatest percentage of variability (7 per cent), followed by a measure of pica, the number of years the child had sucked its thumb, and the mother's smoking habits (See Table 6.2). This sort of detailed study is vital for the identification of the multiple social factors likely to increase lead risk by their interaction since it is clear, as the 1983 Royal Commission Report concludes, that 'a variety of factors (such as home and personal cleanliness, the age and condition of paintwork in the home, playing in the street and eating with fingers) are often associated in socially disadvantaged children, thereby increasing their intake of lead ...'.

Table 6.2: Variables or Measures Correlating Significantly With Tooth Lead Level

	Tooth lead level	
Variable or measure	Absolute (r)	Adjusted (r)
Family cleanliness scale	0.26	0.27
Peeling paint	0.22	0.24
Mother's smoking	0.19	0.18
Pica	0.16	0.16
Play space	0.16	0.14
Proximity to waste ground, demolition or building sites	0.13	0.14
Diet type	0.12	0.12
Thumbsucking (current frequency)	0.12	0.11
Relationship with baby	−0.12	−0.11
Type of pipes used for drinking water	0.10	0.11
Thumbsucking (length of history)	0.10	0.10
Proximity to industrial premises, factories, etc.	0.10	0.10
Age of housing	0.10	0.10

Source: Smith *et al.* (1983), p. 22

Race

The NHANES II surveys found a consistent difference in blood lead levels between black and white people in the population as a whole and within most subgroups. Across both sexes and all ages black people had significantly higher mean blood lead concentrations than whites and the influence of race was particularly pronounced for young children (aged 6 months to 5 years) where the overall mean difference in blood lead levels was about 6 µg/100 ml. This 40 per cent mean difference decreased to 20 per cent in the 6-17 year age group and to 10 per cent in adults.

The black/white difference in blood leads persisted across the three income groups, although it was less pronounced in the $15,000 or more per annum group. The difference also persisted across dwelling-place — comparisons of people living in cities with more than one million inhabitants with those living in smaller cities and with country-dwellers showed that black people had consistently higher mean blood leads, although the number of rural black people examined was low. In addition, the proportion of children with blood lead levels over the CDC cut-off point for unduly high body lead burden of 30 µg/100ml is significantly higher for black than for white children in all three dwelling places. In the inner cities the difference is approximately fourfold with 4 per cent of white children compared with 15.2 per cent of black children requiring medical follow-up (See Figure 6.10).

The UK EEC study was less well suited for the investigation of racial differences in blood leads. Most samples included very small proportions of non-whites and the data showed no consistent evidence of differences between mean blood lead levels of whites and of adults and children in either the West Indian/African or Indian/Pakistani/Bangladeshi racial groups. In fact, in a small sample of Asian children compared to a group of white children living in Tower Hamlets (DOE, 1983), the Asians had the lower mean blood lead level by 1.4 µg/100ml.

In contrast, a larger population study of pre-school children attending playgroups and nursery schools in Birmingham (DOE, 1982) reported that blood lead values in excess of 35 µg/100ml were found almost exclusively in children of Asian parents. This

Figure 6.10: Mean Blood Lead Levels of Black and White Children in the US in Relation to Degree of Urbanisation

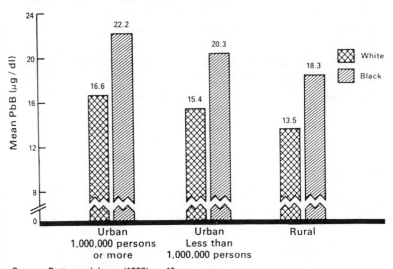

Source: Rutter and Jones (1983), p. 40

result seems less surprising given that Asian homes may contain additional lead sources such as lead-containing cosmetics.

It is increasingly clear that many racial differences are due to social differences between the racial groups under study. In the NHANES II survey for example, it is probable that the blood lead differences observed between black and white children are attributable partly to uncontrolled factors such as play area and age of housing. The majority of black children between 6 months and 5 years old lived in inner city areas and of these, 43 per cent compared to 22 per cent of white children from the same areas were from households near the poverty threshold (family income $\leqslant \$ 6000$ p.a.). In the US, the inner cities have most of the older housing which is often in a dilapidated state and is more likely to be occupied by poorer people — so a larger proportion of the urban black people, particularly children, is likely to be exposed to more environmental lead. Nevertheless, a consistent mean difference between black and white children within all three urban-rural groups indicates that the effects are not completely explained by housing type, although the number of rural black children is small.

Smoking and Drinking Habits

Studies from a number of different countries concur in finding that smoking is associated with higher blood lead levels. The WHO screening survey (Vahter, 1982) found on average that the median blood lead levels for adult smokers in 10 countries were 1.1 times higher than those of non-smokers. In the UK EEC surveys results for both sexes showed that blood lead levels for heavy smokers (more than 20 cigarettes per day) were consistently 10-15 per cent ($1-1.5\mu g/100ml$) higher than in non-smokers. Of greater relevance to children is the finding of the Institute of Child Health Study (Smith *et al.*, 1983) that there was an association between the mothers' smoking habits and the child's tooth lead levels, suggesting that passive smoking can also influence body lead burden.

The results for alcohol consumption are less conclusive but indicate that for men and women who drink 'some' alcoholic drinks, blood lead levels are higher than those of non-drinkers.

Chronological Trends in Blood Lead Levels

Seasonal Variation

There are almost no published data on seasonal trends in blood lead levels in children though it is a well-known observation that cases of chronic lead poisoning peak in summer (Hunter, 1977). Neither the UK EEC survey or the NHANES II study were designed to look at seasonal variations in blood lead levels. The NHANES II survey continued from Spring 1976 to Spring 1980 but as pointed out in their report (Annest *et al.*, 1982) the collection of blood lead specimens took place for logistic reasons during summertime in northern states and during the winter in the south. Any seasonal effects would therefore be confounded with those of geographical location and degree of urbanisation of place of residence. Mean blood levels were observed to be generally higher during the summer months than during the winter months.

Both UK surveys (in 1979 and 1981) took place in most areas over a relatively limited time period during spring. There was no significant variation observed in overall mean blood lead concentration from month to month. The 1979 survey however, included a high lead risk sample of mothers and babies in Glasgow whose blood leads had been collected over a slightly longer period (DOE, 1981). Higher mean blood lead concentrations were observed during the summer and autumn, though the results must be interpreted with caution because of the very small number of samples collected in some months.

One of the few published reports on seasonal trends in a prospective study of children is that of Hammond *et al.* (1983). They have characterised the blood lead profiles of high lead risk urban children aged 0-2 years at three monthly intervals. They present figures for the temporal trends in blood lead levels for infants in four age groups — 10 days old, 3 months old, 6 months and 9 months (See Figure 6.11). The plotted values are derived by regression techniques from the blood lead data of all children at the designated age determined at the specified month of the year. They show that lead levels in infants generally reach a minimum during the spring months — February, March and April and a maximum during August, September and October. The seasonal trend becomes more pronounced with increasing age up to nine months after which, according to the authors, it falls away. They

Figure 6.11: Seasonal Fluctuations in Blood Lead. Each point is derived by regression techniques from blood lead data of all the children at the designated age, determined in the specified month of the year

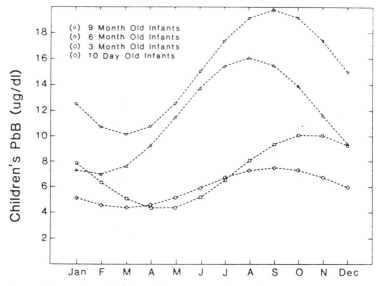

Source: Hammond *et al.* (1983), p. 266

suggest that this is due to increased exposure to extraneous sources of lead since the seasonal influence is seen predominantly in the children living in homes with low hazard for lead (public housing and rehabilitated housing) who have lower mean blood lead levels.

Hunter (1977) suggested that the seasonal difference was partly due to physiological reasons (the increased absorption of lead from the gastrointestinal tract in higher solar radiation) and partly to increased aerosol lead concentrations due to drier weather and higher traffic flow in summertime. To this could be added an increased exposure to external lead sources such as roadside dust in summer when even young children would be likely to spend more time outdoors. The child's increasing activity, together with seasonal variation in dietary lead levels could account for the increasing variation up to 9 months old.

Longitudinal Time Trends

Many different long-term studies of blood lead levels in adults suggest that blood lead levels world-wide have fallen substantially during the last few years. These include the UK EEC surveys, several Welsh studies and the NHANES II survey. It is important to emphasise that none of the studies involved serial blood lead sampling, they were based on a number of different (usually randomly selected) groups of subjects examined at different times. This makes the consensus across studies particularly impressive.

Although the 1979 and 1981 EEC surveys in the UK were of different sample design and therefore produced results which are not strictly comparable, broad comparison of surveys taken within the same local area indicated an overall reduction in mean blood lead approaching 10 per cent (1 µg/100ml) over the two years.

The Welsh data were obtained from eight different surveys based on representative samples of adult women (mostly drawn at random from the electoral rolls for defined areas) conducted at various different times from 1972 to 1982 (Elwood, 1983). Overall the results suggested that blood lead levels in Wales have fallen by over 30 per cent during this period. Two surveys carried out in the same area of Gwynedd, one in 1974 and one in 1982, showed that the mean blood lead level in women fell by at least 37 per cent over this period. Two surveys conducted in the same old lead mining area show a fall of 21 per cent between 1976 and 1981. It is unlikely that either of these decreases is due to changes in water lead since this remained fairly constant, nor to laboratory drift in view of the quality control schemes employed. Elwood suggests that the change is mainly attributable to a decrease in lead intake in food due to an increase in the consumption of frozen, rather than canned foods, together with improved canning and other food preparation methods.

The findings of the NHANES II study are most interesting in comparison to those UK results, since a decrease of 37 per cent in population mean blood lead levels between February 1976 and February 1980 is attributed mainly to a fall in lead in petrol (See Figure 6.12) (Annest, 1983, Annest *et al.*, 1983). The overall mean blood lead level fell from 15.8 µg/100ml in 1976 to 10.0 µg/100ml in 1980. After accounting for the effects of race, sex, age, region of the country, season, income and degree of urbanisation by including appropriate indicator variables in a step-wise (or sequential) linear regression model, a significant (at $P < 0.05$) chronological trend in blood lead levels remained across the whole time period. In contrast, no significant chronological trend was

Figure 6.12: Weighted Mean Blood Lead Values of US Persons from February 1976 to February 1980

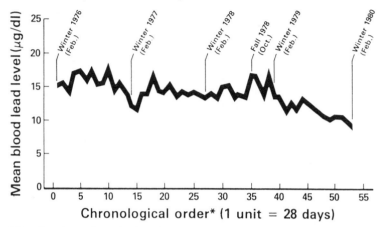

Chronological order* (1 unit = 28 days)

* Based on dates of examination of NHANES II examinees with blood lead determinations
Source: Annest (1983), p. 48

found in the quality control data, indicating that the result was not an artefact of laboratory drift.

After considering and rejecting the possibility that either decreased dietary lead intake or increased public awareness of the lead hazard could be responsible for the observed trend, Annest *et al.* examined their results in relation to the amounts of lead used in the petrol produced in the US over the survey period. Quarterly figures obtained from the Environmental Protection Agency (EPA) showed that the total amount of lead used in petrol production decreased from approximately 53,000 tons to 24,000 tons per quarter from 1976 to 1980. A plot of the overall mean blood lead for six month periods alongside the total lead used in petrol for the same periods indicated a fairly close correspondence between the two sets of figures (See Figure 6.13). Regression of the mean blood lead levels on the EPA petrol lead values and the demographic indicator variables confirmed that in the overall sample as well as within population subgroups defined by race, sex and age, the regression coefficient of the petrol-lead variable was significant at $P < 0.001$. The correlation between blood lead values adjusted for demographic variables and petrol lead at six monthly intervals (Annest *et al.*, 1983) was particularly strong for young white children aged 6 months to 5 years with a Pearson

Figure 6.13: Trends in Blood Lead, Petrol Lead and Dietary Lead in the USA, 1976-1980

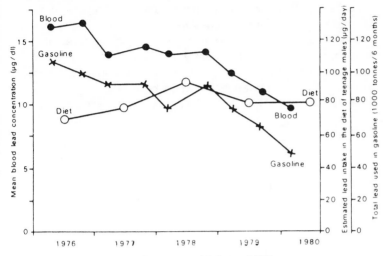

Source: Royal Commission on Environmental Pollution (1983)

correlation coefficient of 0.95 (See Figure 6.14). The researchers concluded that though a strong correlation does not prove cause and effect, the most reasonable explanation for the chronological trend in blood lead values appeared to be the reduction in lead used in petrol production over the same period.

These figures were subsequently subjected to critical reanalyses by interested parties in the petroleum industry (Lynam *et al.*, 1983; Pierrard *et al.*, 1983). After considering these an EPA review concluded that there is strong evidence for the chronological decline in population blood lead levels and that the hypothesis that petrol lead is a causal factor in this decline must receive serious consideration 'in the absence of scientifically plausible alternative explanations' (EPA, 1983). They do, however, caution against using the regression coefficients obtained to quantify the causal effect of petrol lead, and against extrapolation of the relationship beyond the survey period (see also Chapter 14).

In support of the NHANES II results, a recent study by Rabinowitz and Needleman (1983) showed a close correlation between the lead content of all petrol sold in Massachusetts between April 1979 and April 1981 and the concentration of lead in umbilical cord blood from births at a Boston hospital.

Figure 6.14: Average Blood Lead Levels by Six-Month Periods of White Children Six Months to Five Years Old, Plotted against Total Lead Used in Petrol Production per Six Months. The lead values used to compute these averages were preadjusted by regression analysis to account for the effects of sex, income, degree of urbanisation, region of the country, and season. Averages were based on the six-month periods January-June and July-December, except the first and last periods, which covered only February-June 1976 and January-February 1980, respectively

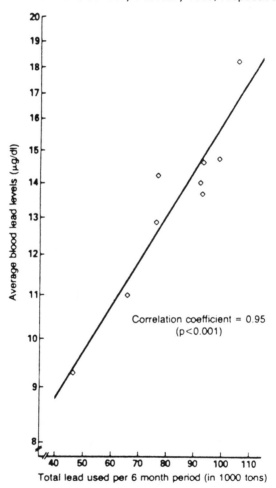

Source: Annest *et al.* (1983)

Though these results for the USA are impressive the petrol lead-blood lead correlation is not necessarily extendable to the UK findings. Until recently the fall in the level of lead in petrol seems to have been balanced by an increase in petrol consumption (DHSS, 1980). Most researchers seem to favour an explanation involving a combination of other factors, such as a fall in dietary lead (MAFF (1982) report a 64 per cent fall in lead in the diet between 1972 and 1980), a decrease in water lead in areas with naturally plumbosolvent water, and the increasing public awareness of lead as a health hazard. Monitoring of the consequences of removal of lead in petrol for population blood lead levels should provide more concrete information with regard to the causal hypothesis.

Conclusions — Correlates and Causes

The evidence derived from the sort of large-scale population studies I have cited here cannot be used to infer causal connections between sources of lead and body lead burden. Nevertheless it is possible, using the cut-off points adoptd by the UK and US studies, first, to identify groups of children at particular risk for high body lead burden, then to use the characteristics of the group to identify the environmental and social factors consistently associated with elevated blood lead.

The NHANES II data indicate that about 4 per cent or approximately 675000 US children of 6 months to 5 years of age have blood lead levels of over 30 µg/100 ml. Among children of this age an estimated 12.2 per cent of black children compared to 2.0 per cent of white children had elevated blood lead levels. The proportion of boys with excessive blood lead level is slightly higher than for girls though the difference is not statistically significant at $P<0.05$. There was a significant decrease in the proportion of children with elevated blood lead levels with increased family income and with decreased degree of urbanisation. The greater proportion of excess blood lead levels in black children held across almost all categories. Though more detailed examination of the data was not possible due to some small cell sizes, other studies have shown that the children most likely to have elevated blood lead levels in the UK are black children living in the central areas of large cities.

In the EEC studies, population blood lead distributions were compared to a set of 'reference levels' formulated in 1977 (See above under 'UK Screening Campaign for Lead'). There were four groups of UK children which exceeded some of these reference levels in 1979. A group of babies in Glasgow exposed to high water lead concentrations — particularly those living in pre-1945 dwellings — breached the two upper reference levels. Twenty per cent of the sample had blood lead levels of over 30 μg/100 ml. Three per cent of a sample of leadworkers' children in Thorpe, Leeds and 6 per cent of leadworkers' children in Chester had blood lead levels of over 35 μg/100 ml; and finally 7 per cent of children living near the Chester lead works exceeded the 35 μg/100 ml level. These latter groups were probably exposed to excess lead-rich dust carried out from the works on clothing and vehicles. In 1981 all these groups were resampled and all met the reference levels, measures having been taken in the meantime to reduce lead sources.

All the adults with elevated blood lead levels were either living in areas with highly plumbosolvent water (Glasgow and Ayr) or had been exposed to specific sources of lead such as old paint (a group in Islington, London).

On the basis of these results, the lead sources most likely to be associated with excessive blood lead levels in children appear to be plumbosolvent water combined with lead domestic piping, and dust lead derived from old paint, or from carry out from lead works. The more pervasive sources of lead, particularly petrol lead, tend not to be implicated as causes of local excessive blood leads but rather in raising the mean overall lead level of a population.

References

Annest, J.L. (1983) Trends in the blood lead levels of the US population — NHANES II 1976-1980, in M. Rutter and R.R. Jones (eds.) *Lead Versus Health*, John Wiley, London and New York.

——, Mahaffey, K.R., Cox, D.H. and Roberts, J. (1982) Blood lead levels for persons 6 months — 74 years of age: United States 1976-1980. NCHS Advancedata No. 79.

——, Pirkle, J.L., Mackuc, D., Neese, J.W., Bayse, D.D. and Kovar, M.G., (1983) Chronological trends in blood lead levels between 1976 and 1980. *N. Engl. J. Med.*, *308*, 1373-7.

Barltrop, D. and Strehlow, C.D. (1982) Cadmium and health in Shipham. *Lancet*, *ii*, 1394.

DHSS (1980) *Lead and Health* Report of the Working Party on Lead in the Environment (The Lawther Report). HMSO, London.

DOE (1978) Lead pollution in Birmingham, Pollution Paper No. 14 HMSO London.

— (1981) European Community Screening Programme for lead: United Kingdom. Results for 1979-1980. Pollution Report No. 10, DOE, London.

— (1982) Blood lead concentrations in pre-school children in Birmingham. A report of the Steering Committee on Environmental Lead in Birmingham. Pollution Report No. 15, DOE, London.

— (1983) European Community Screening Programme for Lead: United Kingdom Results for 1981. Pollution Report No. 18. DOE, London.

Duggan, M.J. (1983) Lead in dust as a source of children's body lead, in M. Rutter and R.R. Jones (eds.) *Lead versus Health*, John Wiley, London and New York.

Elwood, P.C. (1983) Changes in blood lead in Wales 1972-1982, in *Lead in Wales* MRC, Cardiff.

— and Blaney, R. (1983) Blood lead levels on a remote island, *Lead in Wales*, MRC, Cardiff.

Environmental Protection Agency, Appendix 11-D (1983) Report of the NHANES II Time Trend Analysis Review Group, June 15. EPA, N. Carolina.

Hammond, P.B., Bornschein, R.L., Succop, P.A. and Clark, C.S. (1983) Profiles of lead burdens in early childhood. A longitudinal study in a high risk environment, in *Heavy Metals in the Environment, Heidelberg — September 1983* Vol. I, CEP, Edinburgh.

Hunter, J.M. (1977) The summer disease, an integrative model of the seasonality aspects of childhood lead poisoning. *Soc. Sci. Med.*, *11*, 691-703.

Lynam, D.R., Hughmark, G.A., Fort, B.F. and Hall, C.A. (1983) Blood lead concentrations and gasoline lead usage, in *Heavy Metals in the Environment, Heidelberg — September 1983*, Vol. I, CEP, Edinburgh.

Ministry of Agriculture, Fisheries and Food (1982) Survey of lead in food. Second supplementary report. Working Party on the Monitoring of Foodstuffs for Heavy Metals, Tenth Report. HMSO, London.

Pierrard, J.M., Pfeifer, C.G. and Snee, R.D. (1983) Assessment of blood lead levels in the USA from NHANES II data, in *Heavy Metals in the Environment, Heidelberg — September 1983*. Vol. I CEP, Edinburgh.

'*Plwnn Yng Nghymru — Lead in Wales*' (1983) MRC Epidemiology Unit, MRC, Cardiff.

Quinn, M.J. (1983) Factors affecting blood lead concentrations in the United Kingdom, in *Heavy Metals in the Environment. Heidelberg — September 1983*, Vol. I, CEP, Edinburgh.

Rabinowitz, M.B. and Needleman, H.L. (1983) Petrol sales and umbilical cord blood lead levels in Boston, Massachusetts, *Lancet, i,* 63.

Registrar-General's Classification of Occupations (1980) Office of Population Censuses and Surveys, HMSO, London.

Richardson, R.M. (1982) Blood-lead concentrations in three to eight year old school children from Dublin City and rural county Wicklow, *Irish J. Med. Sci.*, *151*, 203-10.

Roels, H.A., Buchet, J-P, Lauwerys, R.R., Bruzux, P., Claeys-Thoreau, F., La Fontaine, A. and Verdwyn, G. (1980) Exposure to lead by the oral and the pulmonary routes of children living in the vicinity of a primary lead smelter. *Environ. Res.*, *22*, 81-94.

Royal Commission on Environmental Pollution (1983) Lead in the Environment Ninth Report, HMSO, London.

Rutter, M. and Jones, R.R. (eds.) (1983) *Lead Verus Health*, John Wiley, London and New York.

Smith, M., Delves, T., Lansdown, R., Clayton, B. and Graham, P. (1983) The effects of lead exposure on urban children; the Institute of Child Health/Southampton Study, *Dev. Med. Child Neurol.*, 25 (Suppl. 47).

Vahter, M. (ed.) (1982) *Assessment of Human Exposure to Lead and Cadmium through Biological Monitoring*, National Swedish Institute of Environmental Medicine and Karolinska Institute, Stockholm.

PART TWO

SOURCES OF LEAD EXPOSURE

Michael R. Moore

Introduction

Although much debate rages and will probably continue to rage around the world about likely means by which man is exposed to lead it should never be forgotten that all lead comes ultimately from the earth's crust and is immutable (see also Chapter 1). It should also be remembered that because of its usefulness to man its future technology will probably match its history. It will continue to be used and will continue to present toxicological problems because of its proximity to man.

When one looks objectively at the origins of lead within the biosphere there are potentially three: lead in soils, lead in air and lead in waters. Each of these will, of course, interact with each other and each represents a very different form of exposure vector.

7 LEAD IN SOILS

Soil lead concentrations normally reflect imperfectly the composition of the parent mineral material with alterations taking place as a function of ageing and increased humus contents of the soil or the degree of mineralisation of the soil. In areas therefore of high mineralisation there is the nearest association with the parent rock and in such areas soil lead concentrations also tend to be highest. In general granitic rocks with a high acid content tend to have higher lead concentrations than basaltic or basic rock (Taylor, 1964; Lockwood et al., 1972; Volobuev and Golomya, 1972; Flanagan, 1973) (Table 7.1). Thus igneous and metamorphic rocks have lead concentrations in the range 7-20 mg/kg (Turekian and Wedepohl, 1961; Vinogradov, 1956, 1962) with similar values in sedimentary rock, but higher values in shales and sandstones of around 10-70 mg/kg (Wedepohl, 1971) and phosphate rock tends to have values that are higher (Sheldon et al., 1953).

Most farming soils or city soils are ones which are non-

Table 7.1: Lead Content of Rock and Soil

Type	Depth (cm)	Concentration (µg/g)
Rocks		
Limestone		8
Shale		20
Sandstone		7
Granite		44
Basalt		15
Lujavrite		45
Syenite		13
Soils		
Mixed Soil (UK)	0-15	57
Earth (Scotland)	3-18	40
	25-84	10
Podzol (Scotland)	0-18	80
	33-48	50
	61-97	30
	102-109	70
Tropical Brown (Cameroun)		127
Hydromorphic (Cameroun)		12

mineralised and concentrations there will range from 2 to 200 mg/kg with most soils being found in the range 5-25 mg/kg (US Geology Survey, 1976). Where concentrations are greater than this, it is almost certain that there has been lead pollution of the soils or that there is increased mineralisation of the soils. This is especially so where ground has been worked for mineral deposits where concentrations as high as 20000 mg/kg have been found (DOE, 1974). In general, however, agreement on the concentrations of lead in soils is poor probably reflecting the very large range of concentrations that have been found. Archer (1977) analysed 752 samples from farms in the UK. Based on his studies the average concentration in the top layer of agricultural soils was found to be 50 mg/kg. It should be noted that soil concentrations of lead appear to vary with depth thus in the upper 20 cm of soil, concentrations will often be fourfold higher than in lower strata (O'Brien *et al.*, 1980) (Table 7.1). The reasons for this are not entirely clear but is thought to be due to both lead accumulation by plants, this lead then being bound in the surface layer as an insoluble complex (Swaine and Mitchell, 1960) and deposition from the air. It should also be noted that because of this industrial and domestic fallout, lead in surface soils is frequently greater next to large cities and close to busy roads (National Academy of Sciences, 1972) and may also be much higher in areas of mining past or present (Davies, 1971). Where such mining has taken place, heavy metal concentrations in plants are raised (Alloway and Davies, 1971). In the USA reports have been made of values ranging from 240 to 540 mg/kg proximal to busy roads and similar figures were found in New Zealand of 180 mg/kg (Ward *et al.*, 1975) but these values fall rapidly and 100 m from the roadside, top soil will have concentrations at baseline levels of around 60 mg/kg. Where soils are undisturbed, the concentrations can become extremely high. In Los Angeles a value was reported of 3350 mg/kg in a city park and in Oakland a city park had mean values of 4270 mg/kg (Wesolowski *et al.*, 1979) whereas in 77 cities in the USA mean lead concentrations ranged from 1640 to 2410 mg/kg (National Academy of Sciences, 1972). Such values probably reflect gross contamination of the soil through airborne deposition of dusts.

Dusts

Street dusts are those materials which collect on paved roads in towns. Concentrations of lead in such dusts are very variable and analysis of them show that they are principally salts of lead with very limited amounts of alkyl lead compound within them (Harrison, 1976, 1979). This reflects the fact that alkyl leads used as anti-knock in automotive fuels are efficiently scavenged by the alkyl halide additives in fuels. Such street dusts are relatively complex materials, the compositions of which are seldom constant. This is because of changes during weathering, the relatively short residence time in the environment and because the residence time is directly related to climate. The build up of street dust is a combination of aerial depositions of dust by gravitational settling and scavenging of dusts by wind and water. Such dusts have been found to contain typically around 2000 mg/kg in US cities (Hunt *et al.*, 1971), 970 mg/kg in England (Day *et al.*, 1975) and 960 mg/kg in Scotland (Farmer and Lyon, 1977). Water scavenging by rain or by snow is relatively efficient but it has been observed that at sites distal to major sources of pollution dry and wet deposition contributes similar quantities of lead. This background of deposition has been calculated to be around 1000 $\mu g/m^2$/year for both the USA and the UK (NAS, 1980). Dusts close to industrial areas particularly the areas involved in lead smelting can be extremely high. We have seen values of lead as much as 25 per cent of the total weight of dust but typical values lie in the order of 1000-50000 mg/kg.

Childhood Exposure

It is generally considered that children are at greater risk of exposure to dust and soil lead both because of their lesser stature than adults and because of poorer hygiene. It is not uncommon for children to indulge in extensive hand to mouth activity where hands are dirty from soil or dusts, to consume sweets which have been dropped on the ground and indeed to eat dusts and soils as part of pica (Duggan, 1983). The Arnhem lead study showed that the most important determinant of blood lead concentrations in children were the levels of lead in soil and dust both indoors and outdoors (Brunekreef *et al.*, 1981). The same study showed that indoor pollution levels were lower than the corresponding outdoor level (Diemel *et al.*, 1981).

It should be remembered that lead in soils and dusts is relatively unavailable biologically. Lead normally reacts with the soil to form insoluble salts. Other ways in which lead is made unavailable biologically is by complexing with organic materials within the soil such as humic and fulvic acids or alternatively by absorbtion of lead into soil minerals. A number of factors contribute to the mobility of lead in soils and because of this it is virtually impossible to predict behaviour of lead within a given soil. Contributing factors are levels of hydration, chemical composition, pH and organic content of the soil. All must be taken into consideration in the assessment of the soil lead content. In addition, analytical techniques for measurement of total lead in mineral materials are far from precise and in many cases the measurements made of lead in soils reflects only that portion of lead taken into solution by acids or by techniques designed to extract the lead. The efficiency of such techniques varies enormously.

Plants

In the investigation of soil contributions to food chains ultimately ending in man, the initial transfer of lead from the soil to plants is of major importance. This is so because plants as primary food-stuffs interface between geological lead and biological lead and because lead in foodstuffs is the primary source of exposure to man. A number of studies have shown that the uptake of lead by plants is limited. In these circumstances it is appropriate to consider the quantity of soluble lead in soils which is available for plant uptake as opposed to total lead in soils. This is by no means a perfect assessment since plant root action will be an important determinant of the bioavailability of lead in the soil to the plant (NAS, 1972). Acidity and low humus content favour lead uptake by plants (McLean *et al.*, 1969; Zimdahl and Skogerboe, 1979). Even after absorption of lead, translocation within a plant is poor and roots invariably contain greater concentrations of lead than parts of the plant above the ground (Motto *et al.*, 1970). The part of plants above ground can of course become surface contam-inated when deposition of lead takes place from the air (MAFF, 1975). This source of contamination could potentially add signif-icantly to lead content of plant foods but becomes less significant to man where these foods are washed and/or peeled (Bryce-Smith and Stephens, 1981). Indeed Ter Haar (1970) concluded that lead content of edible plants was unaffected by increased concentrations of lead in soil from anthropogenic sources.

Natural Radioactive Lead

An interesting means by which one could assess uptake of lead by plants was suggested by O'Brien *et al.* (1980) utilising the presence of natural radioactive lead in the air. Lead-210 with a half-life of 21 years is produced by the decay of Radon-222 and is present in the air in fairly uniform concentrations. A number of assumptions are made in his calculations such as the average value of lead in the air in rural areas being 0.1 $\mu g/m^3$, the annual deposition rate from air in rural areas being 2 $\mu g/cm^2/year$ and the mean concentration of lead in soils being 50 $\mu g/g$. Assuming that and that the mean radioactivity of lead-210 in the air is 0.5 mBq/m^3, the annual deposition rate of lead-210 in the northern hemisphere is 7.4 $mBq/cm/year$ and the estimated average activity of lead-210 in soils is 0.03 mBq/g means that in the air there is a specific radioactivity of 5000 mBq/g, in the depositions from the air 3700 mBq/g with soil specific radioactivity of 600 mBq/g in rural areas. Dietary lead specific radioactivity for lead-210 has been calculated as 530 mBq/g in New York and 860 mBq/g in the UK. This means that the specific radioactivity of these foodstuffs is approximately the same as the specific radioactivity of soil lead but considerably less than the specific radioactivity of lead in the air. This implies that most dietary lead originates from soils presumably through plants and animals and implies further that the residence time of lead in the soil before uptake by plants is at least five times greater than the half-life of lead-210, that is, greater than 100 years. In fact it has been estimated that the residence time of lead in soil in the UK lies between 400 and 3000 years (Bowen, 1975). A consequence of this is that even if all sources of lead exposure were removed immediately, a considerable time would elapse before the benefit of this could be appreciated.

8 LEAD IN THE AIR

Lead in the atmosphere comes from an enormous variety of natural and anthropogenic sources (Nriagu, 1980) (Table 8.1). Where the half-life of lead in soils is relatively long, indeed in some circumstances such as minerals, infinite, the half-life of lead in the atmosphere is short. This is because atmospheric lead is principally particulate and half-lives are therefore determined by the sedimentation velocity which is a function of the mean particle size of these materials. Thus smaller particles, say less than 5 μm will have longer half-lives (Harrison and Laxen, 1981). Ten hours is typical of the residence time of urban and industrial particles, whereas in the troposphere it is of the order of 6-12 days (Nriagu, 1978). Several important factors must be taken into account in estimation of atmospheric lead concentrations. The first is that most techniques used to date to measure atmospheric lead have used filter systems which do not trap the volatile organic lead compounds.

Table 8.1: Sources of Lead Additions to the Atmosphere

	Estimated global emission 10^9g/annum
1. Natural	
Dusts	16
Volcanic output	6.4
Vegetation	1.6
Forest fire	0.5
Sea spray	0.02
Total	24.5
2. Anthropogenic	
Mining	8.2
Primary lead production	31.0
Primary non-ferrous production	45.5
Secondary smelting	0.8
Iron and steel production	50
Industrial uses	7.4
Coal combustion	14
Petrol combustion	273
Waste incineration	8.9
Miscellaneous	10.4
Total	449
	Total emissions 474

Source: NAS (1980)

Such organic lead compounds are more readily absorbed by humans and are therefore proportionately much more dangerous than insoluble particulate material which none the less may be absorbed fairly readily (Baily *et al.*, 1977). Particulate material is most readily absorbed when particle size is small. Although a limited amount of information is available on particle size distribution in the air, it is clear from a number of studies that ageing of lead aerosols results in marked alterations in particle size and chemical composition (Chamberlain *et al.*, 1978). Finally although considerable volumes of evidence are available on atmospheric lead concentrations little is known about deposition rates from the air.

Automobile Exhaust Emission

Despite all this it is clear from current evidence that the greatest source of atmospheric lead pollution is from automotive vehicle emissions (Bryce-Smith and Stephens, 1981) and is particularly high next to busy roads. This source at the current time is diminishing because of the progressive introduction of lead-free petrol or lower lead petrol in the USA (Centre for Disease Control, 1982; Annest, 1983), Japan (Ohi *et al.*, 1981) and in Europe (Sinn, 1981; Department of the Environment, 1983) but still remains a major source of input of lead to the biosphere. Proof of the amelioration of exposure may in fact take many years to be found because of the long half-life of lead in soil and dusts, as was shown in studies of urban pigeons in Tokyo (Ohi *et al.*, 1974, 1981). Lead levels in these birds fell only some years after deleading of petrol had been implemented.

Table 8.2: Alkyl Leads: Properties

	Tetra-ethyl lead	Tetramethyl lead
Chemical formula	$Pb (C_2H_5)_4$	$Pb (CH_3)_4$
Odour	faint, fruity	nearly odourless
Density at 20°C	1.65 g/ml	1.99 g/ml
Vapour pressure at 20°C	0.27 mm Hg	22.5 mm Hg
Boiling point	199°C	110°C
Flash point	85°C	38°C
Solubility in water	0.18 mg/kg	18 mg/kg
Both as clear oily liquids are totally miscible with petrol		

Alkyl Lead

Alkyl leads used as anti-knock in automotive fuels are a combination of a number of compounds, tetramethyl, tetra-ethyl and various mixed alkyl lead compounds (Table 8.2). The recommendations of allowable limits of alkyl lead in petrol vary, although in Europe a consensus seems to have settled on a value of 0.15g/l. After combustion around 75 per cent of lead is emitted from the exhaust as inorganic salts of lead with about 1 per cent of

Figure 8.1: Airborne Lead Emissions from Automobiles During Driving. This diagram shown that the type of emission is highly dependent upon the mode of driving

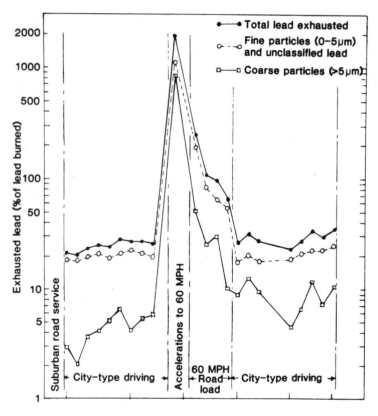

Source: American Chemical Society © Hirschler, D.A. *et al.* (1957) Indust. Eng. Chem. *49*, 1131-42

the alkyl material remaining uncombusted (Harrison and Laxen, 1981), the residual materials being trapped in the exhaust system and engine oil. This does not, however, represent the whole story. A number of factors contribute to variable emissions of alkyl leads in exhausts. In fast motorway type driving, little is emitted, whereas while engines are cold during slow city driving, quantities are considerably greater, as is also the case with two stroke engines (Grandjean, 1983). A similar variation exists depending on the driving mode, of inorganic lead emission. Figure 8.1 shows that the amount of lead emission increases enormously during rapid acceleration but remains low during slow 'city type' driving (Chamberlain *et al.*, 1978; Hirschler *et al.*, 1957). It also shows that there is some variation in the type and proportion of particles emitted during different types of driving, larger particle content increasing during acceleration whereas in normal driving small particles of less than 5 μm were found. It is noteworthy that Chamberlain *et al.* did not find such large particle size in the UK. Small particles are the most hazardous and these predominate in the early phase of exhaust emission. Thus, immediately following combustion primary particulates are as small as 0.015 μm in diameter. These rapidly agglomerate during the ageing process and deposit as dusts.

The Ratio of Natural and Anthropogenic Air Lead

In consideration of 'base line' levels of lead in the atmosphere it is interesting to determine the proportion of these that are a composite of natural and anthropogenic sources. This could be measured through analysis of isotopic composition of the lead and comparing this with isotopic composition of soils in the area under investigation (Ault *et al.*, 1970) and has been done in Italy (Facchetti *et al.*, 1982). Alternatively, it could be measured by consideration of the enrichment factor of lead in an atmospheric aerosol. The enrichment factor is defined as the ratio of the concentration of the lead to that of aluminium in the aerosol divided by the same ratio for the average soil in the area in question, aluminium being chosen as a relatively constant component of soil at high concentration. It is obvious that if atmospheric lead was made up of dust from soil, the enrichment factor would be close to unity. The general finding is, however, that such figures are usually far from unity. Even in areas remote from industrial and urban conurbations, the enrichment factor has been found to be as much as 1000. This is the consistent kind of contamination observed in the work of Murozumi *et al.* (1969) in Greenland and Antarctica, although his interpretation has been questioned (Robinson, 1981). Enrichment factors from natural sources such as the burning of fossil fuels or from volcanic eruption are much lower, in the order of 9 for fossil fuels and 100 for volcanic eruption (Bertine and Goldberg, 1971; Mroz and Zoller, 1975).

Such sources represent the principal 'natural' inputs of lead to the atmosphere, wind-blown particulates being of particular importance which may come from both sea spray and plants, as well as these other sources (NAS, 1980). Concentrations of lead in the southern hemisphere with a much lower degree of industrialisation than the northern hemisphere are lower although concentrations of lead in non-urban zones are equivalent in both hemispheres. In the northern hemisphere baseline levels over seas range between 0.2 and 6.0 $\mu g/\mu m^3$. Whereas in rural areas values range between 50 and 200 $ng/\mu m^3$ (O'Brien *et al.*, 1980) and in the southern hemisphere lie around 20 $\mu g/\mu m^3$. In an attempt to control such exposures to man various legislative moves have been made to limit air lead concentrations. In Europe, a directive of the Commission of the European Communities states, 'an annual mean level of not more than two microgrammes Pb/m^3 in urban residential areas and areas exposed to sources of atmospheric lead other than motor vehicle traffic' and 'a monthly median level of not more than eight microgrammes Pb/m^3 in areas particularly exposed to motor vehicle traffic' (EEC, 1975b). Similar regulations have been formulated in the USA (EPA, 1979).

Automobile Exhaust

Typical of the input of lead into the atmosphere from automobile exhausts, it has been found that in urban air, the concentration of lead can exceed 2 $\mu g/\mu m^3$ in large cities (DHSS, 1980) and very high values have been found during rush hours in major American cities (38 $\mu g/m^3$) (WHO, 1973) and also in South Africa (28 $\mu g/m^3$). On motorways lead concentrations are also high but are much influenced by wind direction and velocity (Figure 8.2). In contrast to this in remote sites, values as low as 1 $\mu g/m^3$ are not unusual and indeed could be considered to be representative of areas such as the North Pacific and Indian Ocean. Since Patterson (1965)

Figure 8.2: Air and Dust Lead Concentrations Proximal to a Busy Motorway. This demonstrates the profound influence of meteorological factors, especially wind, on the distribution of lead

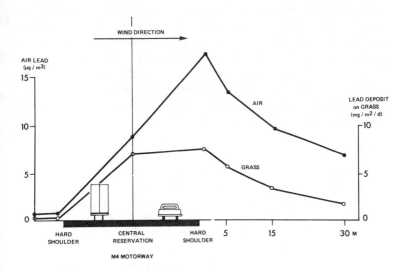

Source: Chamberlain *et al.* (1978)

calculated that the natural concentration of lead in air is 0.6 µg/m³ this implies that a considerable quantity of lead, even in remote areas is of anthropogenic origin.

Fossil Fuel Combustion

Fossil fuel combustion is a major contributor to lead in air. Although most lead concentrates on the ash during combustion such ash does not remain static at the site of combustion but is in the large part carried upward by the plume of hot air and smoke (DOE, 1974). This rate of loss of ash depends on the hot air velocity within the chimney. The greater the velocity the greater the amount of ash carried away from the fire. In major power stations loss of fly ash due to rapid chimney velocities is great and controls have to be introduced to arrest the ash before it is carried away in the atmosphere. Modern stations use electrostatic precipitators with relatively high efficiency. It has been estimated that emissions from sources in the UK are around 50 metric tonnes per year from burning of coal. Crude oil combustion also contributes to lead in the environment but to a lesser extent than from coal. Emissions from this source have been calculated as 15 tonnes per year in the UK (DOE, 1974).

Current industrial emission of lead is relatively low because of the efficiency of control on emission. However, where either primary or secondary smelting of lead is taking place or where lead is being used in the construction of batteries or manufacture of anti-knock compounds, there will be considerable emission to the atmosphere. It has been estimated that this will contribute in total 390 tonnes per annum of which 250 are contributed by smelting processes. Such emissions are principally as lead sulphates and lead oxides (Harrison and Laxen, 1981).

Meteorology

Meteorological and physical features play a major determinant role in the concentrations of lead in the air. This is because by suitable or unsuitable conditions one can prolong the residence time of particulate material in the air dependent obviously on its particle size. Where wind velocities are high particulate material will be more rapidly transported to points distal from the primary pollutant site. Such increases in wind velocity are not exclusively a function of the meteorology but may also be associated with the physical characteristics of the ground over which the air is passing. Thus in city streets running parallel to the prevailing wind there are often increases in velocity because of venturi effects. Such city street effects can also form canyons from which pollution dispersion occurs inefficiently (Struempler, 1976; Cermak and Thompson, 1977). It is also true that increases in rainfall and snowfall will hasten the loss of air-borne particulate material (Grandstaff and Meyer, 1979). This is, of course, not true for alkyl leads which are not in suspension in the air but rather in solution despite high vapour pressures. In this case, the alkyl leads will remain in solution until chemically converted into trialkyl salts or adsorbed onto land mass or other materials. Figure 8.2 shows that on a motorway the deposition of dusts as well as the quantity of lead in air is largely influenced by the wind direction. In conclusion, therefore, every sampling site will have its own characteristics with respect to geography and meteorology and can only be considered individually.

Lead in Petrol (Gasoline)

From all of the foregoing it can be seen that at the current time the primary source of air lead contamination is from additions of lead to petrol. Such additions are no accident. Lead is added to petrol as various types of alkyl lead compound with the primary aim of 'poisoning' this fuel and making it burn more slowly but also more efficiently. The properties of these alkyl compounds are shown in Table 8.2. This is because the basic principle of the internal combustion engine requires that the fuel burns rather than explodes. Indeed the presence of explosions within an internal combustion engine, known as knock, often causes mechanical damage to the engine and usually occurs because the fuel used in the engine has an inappropriate octane number for the engine's compression ratio where octane rating is a measure of the rate of burn of the fuel, or alternatively that the timing of the engine ignition is too advanced. Such internal combustion engines require higher and higher compression ratios to become more efficient and indeed often are required to run at as high a temperature as is possible within the constraints of the cooling system used. Both of these features lead to fuel requirements of higher and higher octane ratings.

It is possible to achieve such high octane ratings by two methods. One is to add greater and greater quantities of burn retardants, such as the lead alkyls or alternatives such as methanol or methyl t-butyl ether. The other is to do this by suitable mixing of the hydrocarbon components of the fuel, the more volatile and short-chain aliphatic hydrocarbons having the lower octane ratings and the more complex cyclic hydrocarbons and branched hydrocarbons having higher octane ratings. At the current time the petroleum industry is achieving octane ratings by combination of these two procedures. The principal advantage of using lead alkyls is that it allows the burn to take place at lower temperatures. This has obvious advantages in the longevity of mechanical components within the engine especially the exhaust valves although this problem may be covered by alterations in engine technology and the use of hardened valve seats.

Because lead is used in petrol and burnt in the engine, it is necessary to add scavengers to fuels to minimise the build up of non-volatile lead deposits. Compounds used for this are ethylene dichloride and ethylene dibromide which promote the formation of volatile lead halides which pass out in the exhaust system but which also contribute to engine wear through acid formation (Aslander, 1977).

There are some economic arguments in favour of maintaining the use of lead alkyls in petrol. Principally it will cost more to produce lead-free petrol at the refining stage. These arguments are generally weak and as has been shown in the USA the actual cost of lead-free petrol is little more than the normal cost of petrol (Bryce-Smith and Stephens, 1981). More important in this respect are the economic costs of continuing to use lead which is associated with a number of deleterious health effects from which there must be a considerable cost to the community from lead exposure.

Such costs need not be exclusively economic but also may be social. Typical of these are the epidemics of solvent sniffing among adolescents. Ordinarily the solvents sniffed are aromatic hydrocarbons but there are numerous instances of petrol sniffing by such children and adults. In such cases, the children are clearly exposed to high concentrations of lead alkyl although this is ameliorated somewhat by the low volatility of these compounds. However, in at least one case an adult was found to have developed lead encephalopathy following petrol sniffing (Law and Nelson, 1968) and skeletal burdens of lead have been found to be raised in such subjects (Eastwell *et al.*, 1983). Such alkyl lead poisoning is a condition not commonly found in the general population being more associated with industrial exposure, either in the factories producing the alkyl lead or as a consequence of working in environments with high alkyl lead concentrations (Beattie *et al.*, 1972) but has also been found in workers using inefficient two stroke engines in chain saws and lawn mowers (Grandjean, 1983) and in petrol vendors (Moore *et al.*, 1976; Kjerschow, 1979). It is noteworthy that in such cases there is a high propensity for the alkyl lead compounds to be found in the lipid components of tissues, pointing to its pronounced effects on peripheral and central nervous function (Beattie *et al.*, 1972; Grandjean, 1983).

The Lead Isotope Experiment

More direct evidence for the influence of air upon man and upon his food has been derived from the isotope lead experiment carried out in Italy during the 1970s and early 1980s. The concept of this experiment was to label petrol on a regional scale with non-radioactive lead of known isotopic composition, this isotopic composition being sufficiently different from the background lead to allow differentiation from local natural sources. Lead isotope 'fingerprinting' of the sources of lead in glass and metallic artefacts has been applied with success to numbers of objects manufactured in old and new world cultures (Farquar and Fletcher, 1980). The ability to carry out this type of analysis depends on two factors. First, the analytical techniques must be sufficiently accurate and there must be an extensive analytical base of isotopic data for potential natural mineralisations. Secondly, significant differences must exist between different sets of isotopic compositions amongst these mineralisations.

The area chosen for this experiment was one to the north of Turin, chosen because Italy has an excess of petrol refining capacity and in consequence does not import either petrol or lead alkyls and because in that country only one firm manufactures alkyl lead as anti-knock. This firm has to buy lead from a state monopoly which could control the source and therefore the isotope composition of lead. The isotope ratio to be examined was chosen as the ratio between lead-206 and lead-207. At the start of the experiment this ratio was found to be 1.18, being supplied from a number of different sources. It was then replaced by lead from the mines at Broken Hill in Australia where the isotope ratio is 1.04.

The results of these experiments suggest that following isotope change there was a dramatic alteration in the ratio of lead-206 to lead-207 in the air which closely paralleled the changes in the petrol/lead ratio (Figure 8.3). Also shown was a change in the isotope ratio in the blood of local inhabitants. In the inner city areas lead concentrations due to airborne lead were calculated as being around 25 per cent of input while in rural areas it lay between 11 and 12 per cent (Facchetti *et al.*, 1982).

This study is not without its critics. Turin is not necessarily typical of other European cities meteorologically or in terms of traffic, and perhaps more importantly, the inhabitants on which the conclusions are based numbered only 35, not selected at random, 13 of whom did not live in Turin. Nevertheless, these results are in very good accord with a number of other experiments in Germany and with calculations of contributions in the UK (DHSS, 1980). Following the alterations of petrol lead concentrations from 0.4-

Figure 8.3: The Lead Isotope Experiment. Changes in the ratios of lead-206 to lead-207 in the Turin area of Italy in the period 1974 to 1981

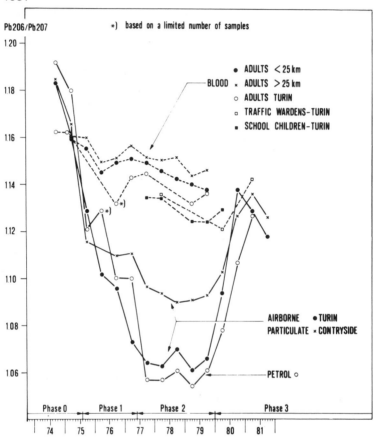

Source: Facchetti *et al.* (1982)

0.15 g/l with a concurrent alteration in the concentrations of lead in the air there were drops in the blood lead concentrations of inhabitants in the city of Frankfurt (Sinn, 1980). Although 25 per cent in inner cities may be due to lead in air, it has been calculated that only 9 per cent of this is taken up by direct inhalation and absorption by the pulmonary route, the residue being ingested as part of the diet. The importance of this is that there are considerable differences in rates of absorption by these two routes as is shown in the chapter on lead absorption by man.

9 LEAD IN WATER

The influence that lead may have in water supplies is conveniently divisible into marine waters and fresh waters. As far as man is concerned the principal source of exposure must inevitably be from fresh water but any point increases in lead concentrations in marine or fresh waters will be reflected in increases in aquatic food source lead concentrations and consequently secondarily in the exposure of man to lead (Pagenkopf *et al.*, 1974; Ray, 1978; Settle and Patterson, 1980).

Seas and Oceans

The bulk of salts in seas which include lead salts arise from long-term concentration of primary fresh water lead. Historically lead input to natural water supplies was determined exclusively by weathering and solution from areas of natural lead mineralisation together with limited deposition from the air. For this reason water pH is of primary importance because it dictates the ability to dissolve salts from such mineralised sources. The more acid the water the greater its ability to dissolve lead. In more recent times lead input into natural water supplies is incremented by atmospheric deposition onto water surfaces. Such deposition does not automatically mean that the lead will go into solution in the water source and indeed it is unlikely that more than a proportion of such material is dissolved. In seas bounded by industrial land masses such as the North Sea it has been estimated that more lead enters the sea by aerial deposition than is input from other water-borne sources (Carter, 1976). Such other water-borne sources are principally river and stream input into marine bodies, which are influenced not only by the type of effluent discharge to the streams such as sewage and industrial waste but also by the absorptive and chemical changes that may take place during the passage of such material to the sea. Salts and muds often bind considerable quantities of lead which in the short-term will remain 'in situ' and even after discharge to the sea, lead bound to suspended material in the water will eventually end up in marine deposits (Harrison

147

and Laxen, 1981). Such lead is unlikely to be directly bioavailable to primary food sources. It is on the basis of lead measurements in such sediments that one finds much of the evidence for increases in lead use and dispersion in the past century (NAS, 1980).

One can calculate that the residence time of lead in the ocean is around 400 years overall (Goldberg *et al.*, 1971) but that the residence time of dissolved material in the surface layer of the water is much shorter, in the order of one year (Turekian, 1977), the removal of lead being due to adsorption onto particles which sediment to the bottom of the ocean (Craig *et al.*, 1973). It has been calculated that the anthropogenic input rate of lead is around 300 000 tonnes per year of which about 60 000 tonnes is soluble. Input from natural sources has been calculated as being 113 000 tonnes per year of which only 13 000 tonnes are soluble (Elias *et al.*, 1975). Current input of lead, therefore, to the oceans of the world of non-natural sources is four times greater than the natural flux. On the basis of his calculations Patterson concluded that the concentrations of lead in surface ocean waters have increased by 0.05 µg/l as a function of industrial pollution (NAS, 1980).

Trophic Chains

In consideration of the role that lead in different forms of water supplies can play upon lead absorption in man, it is of interest to look at aquatic trophic chains to consider the means by which lead may be transferred from bottom sediments and indeed from waters to fish or other organisms that might subsequently become part of the human food chain. A number of techniques have been used to investigate this utilising either artificial ecosystems or separate group measurements in fish typical of their section of the trophic chain. The work of Leland and McNurney (1974) showed a decreasing bioaccumulation of lead the higher the organism involved. Thus, primary producers living in bottom silts had the highest concentrations of lead whereas invertebrates and verte-brate fish lay in intermediate groupings and predatory fish in the lowest grouping of lead concentration. This would be expected since all living organisms only absorb a proportion of the minerals presented to them as part of their food chain and in consequence the higher in a food chain a species lies, the less lead is presented to it and the less lead consequentially it will absorb and retain within its body. The work of Vighi (1981) supported this and showed in addition that as far as fish are concerned, food is the primary factor responsible for lead accumulation, water lead concentration being of lesser import. The actual chemical form of the lead in the trophic chain will of course be of importance and although most lead is inevitably inorganic lead, a small proportion is organic since bacterial methylation of lead has been demonstrated (Wong *et al.*, 1975; Silverberg *et al.*, 1976). Such organic lead will have different routes and rates of absorption to the inorganic material.

Soil and Road 'Run Off'

Water lead concentrations are also influenced by automotive exhaust output. Lead from this source is cleared by both precipitation and run-off from the soil and streets into the hydrosphere. Only a proportion of this material will, however, go into solution and the rest is likely to remain in sediment or in soils with relatively long residence times.

Roads and motorways are the most important source of lead in urban run-off. It has been calculated that from a major urban motorway the average run-off lead is 190 g per day, values being higher in winter than in summer (Hedley and Lockley, 1975). Only a small proportion of this lead is due to contamination of salt used on the roads for de-icing. Thus the total amount of lead discharged in urban areas would depend on the percentage of paved area and traffic density and has been calculated as 0.2-0.3 g per capita per day in urban USA (Bryan, 1974). This type of highway run-off will also contribute enormously to lead concentrations in rural water courses where such water courses are proximal to roads. The predominant source in rural areas, however, must inevitably be from weathering from parent rock and from wash off from soils. In periods of increased rainfall the increases of water flow rate in water courses will mobilise particulate material with consequent increases during rain storm in quantities of transported lead. In these circumstances the greatest increases in lead content will usually occur at the time of maximal rate of change of flow presumably reflecting the ability of the faster flowing waters to move small particulate material. In addition to water passage in water courses, there is also a continuous flow of water from the surface to bed rock to maintain ground water supplies. Such ground waters are generally of lower lead content than might have been expected from initial lead concentration either in the top layers of the soil or rain water. This is because of the filtration and immobilisation process that takes place in the upper layers of soil especially where such upper layers of soil have a high humus content.

Drinking Water

Water as humans drink it, suffers enormously from having to pass through distribution systems (McFarren *et al.*, 1977). Most reservoir supplies of water throughout the world have relatively low concentrations of lead (WHO, 1977). Some treatment of water does take place especially in modern industrialised societies. Principal amongst these is chlorination to provide water of a satisfactory bacteriological quality. Chlorination unfortunately also tends to increase the acidity of water, and acid waters are more capable of dissolving lead and indeed other metals from distribution systems. It has been shown in a number of studies that the lead content of water supplies will rise dramatically where soft acid waters pass through lead plumbing systems (Christison, 1844; Weston, 1920; Moore, 1973). Such plumbing systems do not have to be exclusively of lead construction. Lead-soldered joints on copper systems will also provide an unsatisfactory source of pollution and similar soldering in water boilers for alimentary purposes has been shown to cause increases in water lead content (Reed and Tolley, 1973; Stegavik, 1975; Wong and Berrang, 1976; Lyon and Lenihan, 1977; Moore, 1977). The use of lead stearate for filter in plastics has meant that there has been some experience of uptake of lead from plastic pipes (Heusgem and De Graeve, 1973). This problem is however, minor when compared with that of metal pipes (Packham, 1971). In areas throughout the world, with this type of soft acidic plumbosolvent water supply, it has been shown that water lead concentrations are greatest where the water has been allowed to stand in the lead distribution system for any length of time (Beattie *et al.*, 1972; De Graeve *et al.*, 1975; O'Brien, 1976). Where waters continue to flow in the distribution system lead concentrations are generally lower but still unsatisfactory (Moore, 1977; HMSO, 1977).

Spring Waters

At the end of the eighteenth century some workers considered spring water to be particularly likely to be associated with lead poisoning. This was indubitably due to the acidity of the water (Christison, 1829, 1845). Instances of this occurred in Keighley and other towns in Yorkshire because of the peat-related rise in acidity, water being collected from Moorland sources (Oliver, 1891). Another instance of a similar type occurred when Louis Phillipe and his family moved to Claremont in England in 1848. The estate had been supplied with water for 37 years from a spring, two miles away, through a lead pipe. The local populace had experienced no problems, but on taking up residence Louis Phillipe and his retinue suffered severely from lead poisoning. On investigation it was found that the spring previously open to the air had been covered with an iron dome which allowed carbon dioxide gas to accumulate and to increase the acidity of the water and hence its plumbosolvency (Weston, 1920).

Lead in Plumbing Systems

The problem of plumbosolvency has been compounded by the frequent use of lead-lined tanks as water storage reservoirs. In Glasgow, for example, before remedial water treatment was introduced, 50 per cent of water supplies taken from homes at random had water lead concentrations exceeding 100 µg/l. The majority of these exceeded this by an appreciable amount. It was not uncommon for an individual sample to contain greater than 1000 µg/l especially where a lead tank was present. The water supply at that time had a pH of 6.3 (Richards and Moore, 1982). Only 45 per cent of homes had lead concentrations in random daytime samples of water, of less than 100 µg/l and the mean lead concentration was 244 µg/l with values rising as high as 2000 µg/l. Studies at that time showed that three factors were involved in influencing the uptake of lead by the water. The principal one was the pH of the water, acidic pH being a primary determinant of water plumbosolvency. Also involved, however, were water temperature and type and age of plumbing. The higher the temperature of water, the more lead it dissolved and it was found that mixed metal plumbing systems where lead piping was joined into copper piping, the electrochemical action would also increase plumbosolvency (Moore, 1973, 1983).

Figure 9.1: The Influence of Change of pH on the Plumbosolvency of Lpoch Katrine Water, (Where pH is Maintained at a Value of Around 8 the Rate of Solution of Lead from Lead Plumbing is Minimal)

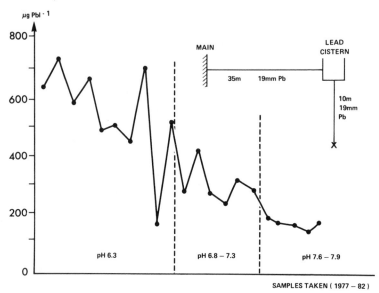

Water pH Correction

Following these initial findings studies indicated that the pH of the water supply could be increased by the addition of lime. Other techniques which could have been used would have been the addition of sodium hyroxide (Karalekas *et al.*, 1977). On this basis a fully automatic closed-loop lime-dosing system was installed at the holding reservoirs for the city of Glasgow and lime additions made to increase the water pH from 6.3 to 7.8 (Richards *et al.*, 1979). This improved the situation dramatically (Figure 9.1). Of random samples 80 per cent now had water lead concentrations of less than 100 µg/l. However, it was observed that in areas distal to the treatment works, the pH value of the water had again fallen to figures less than 7. In consequence, slightly more lime was added to increase the pH further to a value in excess of 8.5. It was then found that at least 95 per cent of random daytime samples had lead concentrations of less than 100 µg/l.

Phosphate

Unsatisfactory samples were, however, still obtained from dwellings with long lengths of old lead piping and from dwellings where the kitchen tap was supplied from a lead-lined tank. In many parts of Scotland it was common practice at the end of the nineteenth century and indeed through into the early twentieth century, to include a lead-lined storage tank to supply water for domestic purposes (Goldberg and Beattie, 1972). This allows not only for a large surface area of lead to be in contact with water for long periods of time but it also allows the water to absorb greater quantities of carbon dioxide from the atmosphere which depressed water pH and from such systems lead concentrations lay between 150 and 350 μg/l. Calculations that were carried out showed that the presence of inorganic phosphate in the water supply would further reduce the solubility of lead by buffering the pH of the water supply. When phosphate was added to the water supply it was found that large concentrations of phosphate were removed from the system by the cast iron mains distribution system so that at the time the water reached the reservoir the phosphate which initially started at 2000 μg/l had fallen to 5 μg/l in the homes. Concentrations of lead in water samples obtained from these dwellings prior to phosphate additions, were high but after phosphate addition contained less than 25 per cent of the lead present before dosage commenced. This meant that samples in areas which previously contained in excess of 100 μg/l fell to a mean lead concentration of 21 μg/l thus putting the values well within the current EEC limits of lead in water (50 μg/l) for domestic purposes (EEC, 1975a). Concurrent with these changes alterations were observed in the mean blood lead content of women living in Glasgow and subjects studied in the town of Ayr (Figure 9.2) (Moore *et al.*, 1981; Richards and Moore, 1982).

The EEC limits are formulated on the principle that average levels of lead in tap water provide less than 10 per cent of the overall daily exposure to lead. The World Health Organization estimated that the natural content of water suitable for alimentary use from lakes and rivers worldwide lay between 1 and 10 μg/l although these levels could be higher where there was some form of industrial or urban contamination (WHO, 1977). During distribution in plumbing systems, however, there is almost invariably some uptake of lead but water lead concentrations tend to remain

Figure 9.2: The Impact of Water Treatment on Maternal Blood Lead Concentrations. Prior to treatment the geometric mean blood lead was 14.6 µg/100 ml, following treatment 8.1 µg/100 ml

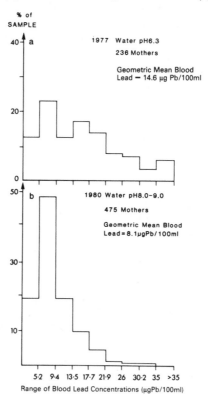

relatively low at less than 10 µg/1 except where circumstances arise where waters are acid, plumbosolvent and where there is lead in the plumbing system. It has been suggested that uptake of lead may occur after the use of kettles which have soldered joints. Indeed in one report from Canada, lead poisoning in an infant was traced to this source (Wigle and Charlebois 1978). This cannot be a major source of pollution since the concentrations of lead in water from kettles has generally been found to be low (DOE, 1982; Lacey *et al.*, 1983).

Water Lead in Diet

If one calculates that a normal human consumption of water is 2 litres per day then the daily intake of lead from this source will supply between 10 and 40 µg/daily. It should be borne in mind, however, that this use of raw waters is not the only means by which lead in water will influence lead intake. Other factors such as adsorption onto foods during cooking processes must be taken into account (Berlin *et al.*, 1977; Moore *et al.*, 1979; Smart *et al.*, 1981). In making many of these calculations on the likely amount of lead ingested it is important to remember that not all ingested material is actually absorbed. Although little is known about the absorption of fine particles of lead from the gastrointestinal tract it has been shown that a considerable proportion of tap water lead exists in particulate or colloidal form rather than in solution. (Harrison and Laxen, 1980). Around 10 per cent of lead is thought to be typical for the amount of lead absorbed by adults but this is considerably influenced by a number of factors such as whether or not the stomach is full and the presence of elements such as calcium, phosphorus and many others in the diet.

Duplicate Diet Study

Valuable guidance on acceptability of the 50 µg/l limit was given by the Duplicate Diet Study carried out in Glasgow in 1979 subsequently repeated in Ayr in 1981 (DOE, 1982; Sherlock *et al.*, 1982; Lacey *et al.*, 1983). The principal aim of this study was to offer guidance on allowable concentrations of lead in drinking water. Many assumptions have to be made in doing this but it is possible on the basis of given standards for blood lead to achieve an upper limit lead concentration in water. Perhaps the principal assumption is that one works on the fairly arbitrary limit of 30 µg/100 ml for blood lead which should not be exceeded in more than 10 per cent of a given population group (Commission of the European Communities, 1977). Because this is a blood standard it would not be valid to translate this into a water standard simply by interpolation in the relationship between means. Especially since there is some doubt about the exact form of the relationship whether linear or non-linear (Moore *et al.*, 1977; DOE, 1982). It is necessary to produce a more complex argument which will take into account population variability. One approach is to calculate the concentration which, if received uniformly by the whole population, would ensure an upper 90 percentile of 30 μg/100 ml for blood lead, that is no more than 10 per cent of the population would have blood leads greater than 30 μg/100 ml. The Duplicate Diet Study provided information which allowed an approximate attempt at such calculation for bottle-fed children (Lacey *et al.*, 1983). To do this one can estimate the upper 90 percentile in terms of the model described by the linear equation:

Figure 9.3: The Estimate of the 90 Percentile Grouping in Children in the City of Glasgow Aged Between 10 and 13 Weeks Who Use Bottle Feed. The graphs show that to comply with the European Community (EC) reference level of blood lead of 30 μg/100 ml, water lead concentrations must be below 70 μg/l. This graph is calculated on a linear approximation of the curvilinear relationship between exposure and blood lead

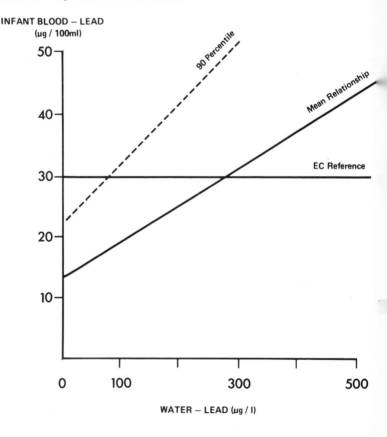

INFANT BLOOD – LEAD
(μg / 100ml)

90 Percentile

Mean Relationship

EC Reference

WATER – LEAD (μg / l)

$$Z_i = B (X_i + A/B) E_i$$

where X_i is the water lead concentration and Z_i is the blood lead concentration of the ith subject in the study and A and B are constants relating to the equation and log E is normally distributed. These calculations show that at the 90 percentile level, the standard of 100 µg/l for water lead might not be low enough to ensure compliance with the requirements for blood lead (Figure 9.3). However, a water lead standard of 50 µg/l as the mean concentration of lead in ingested water, should ensure compliance with a *small* margin of safety. These calculations were made for babies fed with bottled water and strictly speaking babies in the city of Glasgow. Since babies represent perhaps the most affected section of the population, in respect of water lead exposure, this is of course showing the worst case and if these fit within the recommendations then it is likely that other sections of the population will also do so. It should be noted also that for children of the age considered in that study, the value is equivalent to an upper limit to dietary lead intake of 50 µg/week/kg body weight.

There are those, however, who would argue that this does not provide a sufficient margin of safety since blood lead concentrations as low as 30 µg/100 ml have been associated with deleterious effects in humans. The argument presented here can, however, be applied to lower levels of blood lead concentration. There is, however, a high degree of consensus in respect of the acceptable levels of lead in water formulated by various regulatory agencies throughout the world (EEC, 1975a; EPA, 1976; WHO, 1982). The greatest problem that has beset regulatory limits in this respect has been that all have been derived from relatively arbitrary standpoints and in no case is there any degree of equivalence between these limits. The current calculations provide a means of standardisation of these measures.

10 LEAD IN FOOD

When one turns away from the primary origins of lead to which man may become exposed, there are a number of exposure vectors which should be examined as means of input to man. The major vector in this respect is lead concentration in the diet which includes food and water and the contribution to these by lead in the air. There are in addition a number of minor factors that should be taken into account such as lead absorption through the skin and a host of dietary and non-dietary factors which have been implicated in causing lead poisoning in man. It is now generally accepted that, for the majority of the population, alimentary lead exposure is the primary means by which man is exposed to lead and it is by this route that the majority of the lead in the body is absorbed (DHSS, 1980). Less certain are the routes by which the diet becomes exposed to and contaminated by lead and the relative proportions of input from the air, the soil and the water. The problem in differentiating between these different origins is that lead uptake by foods and deposition on foods can be extremely variable and may also be part of a decreasing food chain.

The effects that lead concentration in the air will have upon lead concentrations in food are diverse. It may firstly act directly on the foods, it may pass into soil and thus be taken up by vegetation used either as a primary food source or as fodder for animals and finally it may also be deposited and dissolved in waters and thus be taken up by fish or by increasing concentrations of lead in the water supply acting directly upon man or through uptake into foodstuffs during food preparation.

Most studies carried out of lead absorption have been unable to differentiate between the different sources of lead in foodstuffs and relative intake by alimentary and pulmonary absorption. In most cases pulmonary absorption has been derived by difference as that proportion unaccounted for by lead concentrations in food or in water. This was the approach taken in the Duplicate Diet Studies carried out in Glasgow and Ayr (DOE, 1982; Sherlock *et al.*, 1982; Lacey *et al.*, 1983).

Canned Food

Apart from the obvious sources of lead exposure from the environment and from the air, contamination of lead in foodstuffs may also occur as part of the cooking process or part of storage of the foods. There is clear evidence that canned food in soldered cans becomes contaminated especially where the food is acidic and there is also evidence to show that during the cooking process foods will absorb lead from the cooking medium and from the cooking utensils (MAFF, 1972; Shea, 1973; NAS, 1980; DHSS, 1980).

The standard three-piece soldered can has seen little alteration in its construction since the 1920s. These are produced by rolling tin-plate into a cylinder and soldering the edges together at the overlap. Lead solder is normally used since tin solder is so much more expensive, although this was used for baby foods. It is possible to make the can by welding but this process is slower and therefore not favoured by industry. The alternative to such cans are two piece ones which may be constructed of tin plate or aluminium, by forcing of a 'cup' of metal through a die or 'redrawing' it. Cans present two main sources of lead in food. The first is from the solder joining the sides of the can since this may flow into the can interior. The second is from the tin plate itself, although this is governed by a British Standard to contain no more than 0.08 per cent lead. Nevertheless, highly acidic foodstuffs like plums and apples can leach lead from such plate. This may be avoided by lacquering the inside of the can. It has been estimated that between 10 and 40 per cent of dietary lead can come from cans and that if the proportion of canned food rises from the average of 6.3 per cent of total food intake to 10 per cent then contribution could be as high as 60 per cent (MAFF, 1983). It is for this reason that it has been recommended that limits for lead in canned food be dropped from the current limit of 2 mg/kg to 1 mg/kg as is applicable to fresh food. It has been recognised that this requires some alterations in canning technology but the policy of all responsible manufacturers now seems to be towards construction of welded cans which will be complete by 1985.

The influence that canned food will have on diet is a problematic one. Not only because the amount of lead uptake from soldered cans is extremely variable but also because the relative quantities of canned food used varies enormously from house to house. The Ministry of Agriculture Fisheries and Food (MAFF, 1983) has calculated that canned food will contribute about 15 per cent of the total dietary intake of lead. This is only so for foods destined for adult use. Infant feeds may not by the Lead in Food Regulations of 1979 in the UK have a content of lead greater than 200 µg/kg. In consequence manufacturers do not use lead in the manufacture of cans for infant foods.

Dietary Assessment

Duplicate Diets

Dietary lead intake may be assessed by one of two methods. In the first and perhaps the most satisfactory method, duplicate diets are taken from a number of representative subjects and the lead concentrations in the duplicate diet measured whilst at the same time the subjects' lead status is assessed through blood lead concentration and various other secondary measures such as blood protoporphyrin or erythrocyte aminolaevulinate dehydratase. A number of such studies have been carried out in past years. Those by the Ministry of Agriculture Fisheries and Food in the UK carried out over one week in adults and in children have shown that the dietary intake varied between 21 and 330 µg/day with an average value of 75 µg/day. In children the range of values is very much higher especially where the children examined are younger than 6 months and in whom a major proportion of the diet is milk feed. This is because those children fed on milk have a larger proportion of their diets supplied as water than at any other time in life and in consequence dietary lead content is largely influenced by the water lead content. Large variations in water lead are reflected in the relatively greater variations in dietary lead. The problem is compounded by the fact that those children that are breast fed will generally have very much less lead in their diet than bottle fed children. This is so because breast milk lead concentrations are approximately the same as serum lead concentrations which are about one-tenth of blood lead concentrations (DOE, 1982; Sherlock *et al.*, 1982; Moore *et al.*, 1982; Moore, 1983). In the worst situations, maternal blood lead can lie between 30 and 40 µg/100 ml. This would give breast milk lead concentrations of between 30 and 40 µg/l. For the general population, however, values are much less than this, nearer 3 µg/l equivalent to 0.45 µg/kg/body weight/day.

Total Diets

The alternative means of assessing diet is through total diet studies. This type of investigation requires measurement of lead concentrations in all dietary substituents. These dietary substituents and the relative composition of them are calculated from information obtained by the National Food Survey and the National Household Expenditure Survey in the UK. From the mean quantities of food purchased and presumably consumed, dietary lead calculations give values in the range 55-366 µg/day with a mean of 113 µg/day (MAFF, 1975). This corresponds well with the calculated figures in duplicate diets and indeed with calculation of intake in the USA and other parts of the world (NAS, 1980; WHO, 1977). No trend in food lead equivalent to that seen in air lead has yet been observed (Jelinek, 1982). This type of measure will tend to overestimate values since in many cases the concentration of lead in the dietary component lies below measurable levels and in such instances the values used are given as limits of detection of the analytical method.

Drinking Water

Lead concentrations in drinking water will increase dietary lead content and are of much greater importance in the calculations of dietary lead intake. A number of studies have shown that if foods are cooked in water such foods tend to take up lead from the water supplies, a concentration effect (Berlin *et al.*, 1977; Moore *et al.*, 1979; Smart *et al.*, 1981). In these studies all forms of vegetables, pasta and meats examined showed significant binding of lead from water. Although washing will remove considerable quantities of external contamination from vegetables, this is more than made up for when water lead concentrations are increased and there is uptake of lead into the matrix of these materials. These calculations show that where water lead concentrations lie around 100 µg/l 50 per cent of the dietary lead intake would come from the water (DOE, 1981) although at lower concentrations of lead in water, the proportion becomes relatively less. This calculation is in complete agreement with the information obtained from the duplicate diet studies in Ayr and Glasgow. Although some foods will obviously gain in lead content as a consequence of these cooking processes, beverages such as tea and coffee will have diminished lead concentrations since in these cases tea leaves and coffee grounds bind significant quantities of lead from the water thus lowering the relative concentration in the beverage.

11 LEAD IN PAINT

There are numerous sources to which man is involuntarily exposed to lead. Lead in paint is the major one of such. There are excellent mechanical and chemical reasons for using lead in paint. As a means of inhibiting corrosion on steel structures and in providing a coating capable of withstanding weathering, leaded paints are favourite for use in the construction and engineering industries. The lead in such paints comes from two sources; from the pigments such as red lead or white lead used to colour the paint and as lead naphthenate and octoate used as driers in oil-based paints. Thus apart from the lead oxide paints many other paints not listed as being leaded contain considerable quantities of lead, between 0.25 and 0.5 per cent in many gloss paints.

Historical Perspective

The level and distribution of lead paint in dwelling units is a complex function of history, geography, economics and individual decorating habits. Prior to 1955 there were no regulations in the USA on the amount of lead in paint and similar lack of control was found elsewhere in the world and it is only after that time that one finds a series of more stringent measures controlling the use of lead in paint. This means that houses built before 1955 have more interior lead painted surfaces. On surfaces within the home the evidence generally is that the concentrations of lead are higher on doors or windows which require frequent refurbishment and for which oil-based paints are usually used. In contrast to this lead content on walls when non-oil based paints are more commonly used tend to be much lower (NAS, 1980). It should also be remembered that in the home there are a considerable number of painted tools, furniture and other items. All of which may contribute to overall exposure. Examples of this are toys and painted handles of kitchen utensils (Hankin *et al.*, 1976; Lin-Fu, 1980).

The commonest source of lead poisoning from lead paint is in the demolition and ship breaking industries (Rieke, 1969). In these circumstances oxyacetylene burning of steel structures coated with

Figure 11.1: Strategies for Abatement of Lead Exposure from Paint

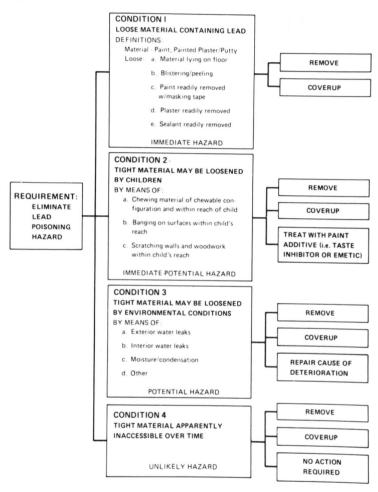

Source: Billick and Gray (1978)

many years of lead-containing paint often provide a highly toxic environment for the workers concerned (Taylor *et al.*, 1974) (Figures 11.1 and 11.2). A good example of this was found during the demolition of a Victorian railway station in Glasgow, St Enochs, when many workers became poisoned during the demolition process (Campbell and Baird, 1977). There are also

Figure 11.2: Strategies for Abatement of Lead Exposure from Paint

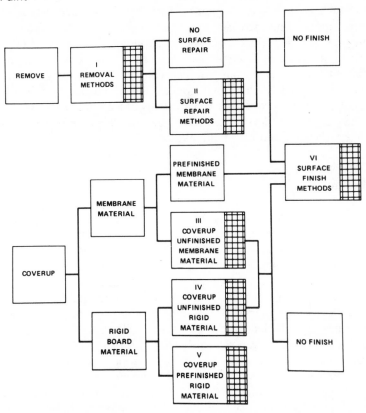

Source: Billick and Gray (1978)

instances of painters both industrial and artistic becoming poisoned (Graham *et al.*, 1981). At the present time, advances in technology mean that the concentration of lead in paint is continuously falling and indeed most paint sold now for domestic use contains little lead. Where greater concentrations are found an EEC directive in Europe demands that warning labels are included on the paint can. The situation in the USA is similar but more bounded by active legislation and indeed by a programme of lead abatement which includes an identification programme (Billick and Gray, 1978) in which lead concentrations in painted surfaces are measured by X-ray fluorescence (Reece *et al.*, 1972). The real hazard from lead in paint usually occurs because of the great longevity of such paints and because eventually as part of weathering such paints come away from the surfaces to which they have been applied and increase the content of lead in dusts and debris proximal to the surfaces (Bogden and Louria, 1975; WHO, 1977). The importance of this type of source can be appreciated from the fact that a very small flake of lead-containing paint may contain over 1 mg of lead, ten times greater than the mean daily intake from all other sources. The bioavailability of lead from such point is generally low, estimated at around one quarter or a half of that ingested (Gage and Litchfield, 1969).

Control

The fact remains, however, that in the UK and in the USA, lead poisoning from paint accounts for the majority of all known cases of lead poisoning, especially in children. The problem is that children frequently indulge in chewing of painted articles. If such painted articles, be it a toy or painted surface within the home contains lead, the children can be exposed to quite enormous quantities of this metal. Parents often consider that re-painting old surfaces is a sufficient measure to make surfaces safe for children. This is not so. Children will easily chew through the newly painted surface and ingest all material both in the upper and lower levels so that a measure like this which would be adequate in adults is quite inadequate for children. Safety is only assured by stripping of surfaces right down to base. The Department of Housing and Urban Development in the USA has outlined a series of strategies that can be followed in the handling of lead-based paint abatement. These are shown in Figures 11.1 and 11.2. The abatement methods that may be applied include the formation of biological barriers such as coatings which have a bad taste or other properties which will stop children chewing them, indicators in the surface material which will cause for example colouration of the lips and mouth when chewed or barriers to absorption such as a use of chelating agents to prevent lead absorption in the body. Physical barriers are a more satisfactory way of controlling the problem. These include various forms of coating which are imperishable, examples of these would be paint and flexible and non-flexible materials such as plastic films or wallboards. The most satisfactory means of all of controlling the lead problem is, however, removal. This may have to go to the point of not just removing the paint from a surface but actually taking away the surface itself, such as the removal of an old door (Billick and Gray, 1978). Such de-leading is itself not without hazard as was found when an urban bridge had lead removed from it in Boston and caused a number of cases of occupational and environmental lead poisoning (Landrigan *et al.*, 1982).

Although this hazard from exposure to lead paints is now clearly defined, there is a general lack of knowledge of just how widespread old-lead painted surfaces are. There is also great disparity in the means by which different governments attempt to control this overexposure. The Federal Government in the USA attempts to do this by a series of rules, regulations and laws. At present (1984) this limit is 0.06 per cent in the dry film. The Commission of the European Communities by directives and the British Government by gentleman's agreements with the industry, sets the limit at 1 per cent in the dry film (British Standard 4310). Which is the most effective remains to be seen but it is obvious that as far as lead paint goes, none whatsoever should be used on toys and it would be preferable to have similar regulations about the home.

Whether or not this could be extended to the engineering industry remains to be seen but it should not be forgotten that if one had a totally de-leaded interior to a home, flaking of outside paint containing lead would contribute enormously not only to the lead content of the dust and soils in the garden next to the home but also effectively, because of wind distribution, to the dust lead content within the home (Gibson *et al.*, 1892).

12 OTHER SOURCES OF EXPOSURE TO LEAD

Other than the obvious exposures to lead associated with its production and use by industry, there are large numbers of other potential environmental sources of lead, some of which might have been suspected and others unsuspected. This chapter attempts to list a few of these.

Printing Inks

In the early investigations of the subject, some workers (Hankin *et al.*, 1973) found a child who had lead poisoning and for whom they could find no obvious source of exposure to lead. They eventually discovered that the child was in the habit of chewing newspapers in which newsprint they found that the lead content could be as high as 3600 μg/g especially on pages containing multi-coloured advertisements. This meant that 22 cm^2 of a coloured magazine page would supply 300 μg of lead. Subsequent investigation by the same authors showed that printed bags and wrappers used for foods could be similarly contaminated with lead salts (Hankin *et al.*, 1974a and b). They pointed out that it was not unusual for newspaper and newsprint to be used in garden mulch or feeding of paper to ruminants by which routes lead would enter the human foodchain although the relative quantities of transfer would be small (Heichel *et al.*, 1974). However, 'spitballs' made by children chewing paper are a definite hazard (Joselow and Bogden, 1977; Hankin *et al.*, 1973).

Cosmetics

Because of its dark lustrous black appearance, lead sulphide has been viewed as a valuable cosmetic compound since antiquity. Lead sulphide is of course a relatively insoluble salt but in its use as a cosmetic, lead is frequently applied not as an insoluble sulphide but as a more soluble compound such as the acetate which in contact with biological materials forms dark grey to black insoluble lead-sulphur compounds. The Romans are reputed to have used this as a basic principle for darkening of their hair by dipping lead combs in vinegar before combing the hair. The lead acetate thus formed enters the complex structure of the hair shaft and in combination with sulphur-containing residues on amino acids of the hair keratin results in the darkening of the shaft. This use of lead represents a toxicological hazard to humans through increased absorption of the metal, which could take place either orally or percutaneously.

Percutaneous Absorption

To date it is generally accepted that the percutaneous absorption of lead is only of importance in the case of organic lead such as naphthenates and alkyl lead compounds (Waldron and Stofen, 1974; Rastogi and Clausen, 1976). As far as inorganic lead salts are concerned, the evidence of absorption is extremely limited. Laug and Kunze (1948) found that lead acetate could be absorbed through the skin of the rat and that there would be an increase in absorption where the skin was damaged. These experiments did, however, relate to rat skin the structure and properties of which are very different to the human skin.

More recently studies have been made of the ability of lead dyes to penetrate human skin. Although one study did find some absorption (Marzulli *et al.*, 1978), it would seem from a study using radioactive lead tracers (Moore *et al.*, 1980) that only very small quantities of lead, between 0 and 0.3 per cent of the applied dose, could be absorbed by this route. The previous study suffered from having assessed lead absorption by measurement of hair content of lead. On principle it would seem unlikely that percutaneous absorption would represent a major source of exposure since at any one time considerable quantities of lead are in continuous contact with the skin either on the clothing, in water or in the air.

Hair

Proteinaceous materials like hair will readily adsorb lead onto their surface from contamination. Moore *et al.* (1980) concluded that the use of lead cosmetics for the hair would contribute around 0.7 µg/week to the quantity of lead absorbed, where the normal quantity of lead absorbed per week would be 266 µg. On the basis of this information and because they could find no evidence for lead being carcinogenic the Food and Drugs Administration of the USA exempted lead from certification subject to a number of restrictions, first, that the lead content should be no more than 0.6 per cent (weight per volume), that it is not used for moustaches, eyelashes, eyebrows or hair on parts of the body other than the scalp and that labelling made it absolutely clear that hands and other parts of the skin should be washed after coming in contact with the product. In particular they noted that it should not be used on broken skin and should be kept out of reach of children (FDA, 1980). In their directive on cosmetics the EEC banned lead except for its uses in hair darkening products (EEC, 1976).

Surma

Such hair dyes are generally aimed at an older section of the population. This is not true of another form of lead dye used in the Indian subcontinent. In that continent lead-containing compounds are used to darken the skin round the eyes of adults but also of children and infants. These compounds, the khols or surmas, were originally formulated from antimony sulphides but because of economic constraints are now commonly made of lead sulphides. Thus although surma has been used by Muslim communities for many centuries, toxicological hazards associated with its use have only recently become obvious. This has been particularly so in the Asian communities in Britain where a number of cases of poisoning have been found (Betts *et al.*, 1973; Snodgrass *et al.*, 1973; Pearl, 1977; Ali *et al.*, 1978; Green *et al.*, 1979) and in Japan and USA where the cosmetics for the face can contain as much as 67 per cent lead (Kato, 1932; Byers, 1959). Official bans were put on the importation of these compounds from the Middle and Far East but it was found that they were often brought in by personal importation following pilgrimages to Mecca or for use by traditional healers in the cities of Northern England. Although younger mothers were often aware of the hazards of these compounds and indeed of the disapproval of European trained physicians, family pressures often resulted in the continuance of their use. The net result was that Asian children as a group tended to have blood lead concentrations higher than their European peers in similar environments. More significantly, a large proportion of the Asian children had blood lead concentrations which lay outside acceptable limits this all being due to surmas which contained greater than 50 per cent lead sulphide.

Unlicensed Medical Products

Lead was first introduced to the Western Pharmacopoeia by Paraceleus in the fifteenth century AD (Singer and Underwood, 1962). It is not long since the removal of lead from the British Pharmacopoeia in which lead and opium pills were prescribed for symptomatic treatment of diarrhoea. These contained 1.6 grains lead acetate and 0.08 grains opium. The availability of these compounds led to an outbreak of lead poisoning in a group of drug addicts in Glasgow when they were dissolved and injected intravenously (Beattie *et al.*, 1977, 1979). Such compounds are no longer available. There are, however, considerable hazards associated with the use of alternative medicines which contain lead either as a primary component or as a trace contaminant. Typical of these are Chinese herbal medications (Lightfoot *et al.*, 1977), aphrodisiacs from the Indian subcontinents, Mexican-American folk medicines (Bose *et al.*, 1983) and a number of other compounds from India (DHSS, 1980). Lead exposure has also been linked with the use of lead nipple shields by nursing mothers (Wilcox and Caffey, 1926) and lead-containing nipple ointment (Holt, 1923).

Ethanol

The 'Dry Gripes'

The association of increased lead absorption with ethanol is one of long standing. In ancient Rome it was accepted practice to sweeten wine with a syrup called Sapa which was prepared in lead pots and contained around 1000 mg/litre lead (Gilfillan, 1965). Even a teaspoonful of this per day would have caused chronic lead poisoning. This practice continued into the middle ages even after the discovery of the aetiology of the lead colics by Glockel (Eisinger, 1977). Legislation such as that of Wurtemberg in 1696, which included the death penalty, attempted to control this but was hampered by inadequate diagnosis and analysis. In the early years of the colonies in America, colic called the 'dry gripes' was described and was eventually associated with rum condensed in lead stills (McCord, 1953). Thus there are two reasons for the association of lead and alcohol. Firstly some alcoholic beverages have increased concentrations of lead in them and secondly, ethanol consumption appears to enhance lead absorption.

Enhanced Absorption and Increased Levels

Of these two the increased quantities in certain beverages is certainly of importance whereas the factor of increased absorption may well be related to a number of features of alcoholism not the least of which is a metabolic acidosis combined with poor nutrition which has been linked with increased gastrointestinal absorption of lead.

The source of increased lead concentrations in some beverages is easy to determine. Illegally distilled (Moonshine) whiskey in the USA and in many other parts of the world often contains lead. The reason lies in the methods of construction of the stills and in the composition of the mash used in the alcoholic fermentation. It was not infrequent for these stills to be made either of lead piping or more commonly disused radiators from cars which have large quantities of lead solder. The mash contains acetic acid which reacts with this lead to form soluble lead acetate which passes with the white lightning (distillate) from the still (Patterson and Jernigan, 1969). As a result of this, lead concentrations of greater than 1000 µg/l have been found in 30 per cent of analysed samples of moonshine whiskey (NAS, 1972). Conventional alcoholic beverages have much lower concentrations of lead. It is not known how much of such illicitly distilled material is made in the USA but it was estimated in 1968 that more than 36 million gallons were produced. In consequence clinical poisoning from moonshine is a far from infrequent occurrence (NAS, 1972).

The normal contribution of lead from alcoholic drinks to the lead content of the diet is relatively low although they may contribute significantly to intake. A pint of beer in Britain will contribute around 10 µg to the daily intake of lead (DHSS, 1980) but more importantly, a number of European wines have very much higher concentrations of lead in them (WHO, 1977). The source of this lead in wine is far from certain but it has been suggested that it is in part due to deposition from automobile fumes (Marletta *et al.*, 1973). Whatever the source, wines have variable lead concentrations but were estimated as being around 250 µg/l in French wines and have found to be much higher in wines from Italy and Hungary (Jaulmes *et al.*, 1960; Nagy *et al.*, 1976). This means that for the normal wine drinker there is a significant input of lead from this source. It has been noted that in countries with high wine intake such as Italy blood lead levels do tend to be marginally higher than in other parts of Europe. More significantly, it means that in alcoholic subjects imbibing large quantities of this material, blood lead concentrations are considerably greater than in normal subjects (Vives *et al.*, 1980; Grandjean *et al.*, 1981). It is difficult to differentiate between increased intake and increased absorption but studies in Britain would certainly seem to suggest that the quantity of intake of alcohol and/or the type of alcohol drunk, be it whiskey or wine or beer, are not related and one must conclude that absorptive factors must play the greater part (Shaper *et al.*, 1982; DOE, 1983).

Smoking

Like alcohol consumption, smoking is thought to play a part in increased lead exposure. There is considerable difficulty in assessing this since most people who drink also smoke and vice versa. There seems little doubt that smoking can contribute to lead concentration particularly where there is increased hand to mouth activity in situations of high lead exposure as an industry (Tola and Nordman, 1977) and also from tobacco grown on fields in which lead arsenate had been used as insecticide (WHO, 1977). Although some authors found little or no difference in blood lead concentrations in relation to smoking habits in most studies there is a trend towards increased blood lead concentrations and it has become clear that independent of alcohol consumption smoking does contribute to blood lead concentrations but to a lesser extent (Zielhuis *et al.*, 1977; Grandjean *et al.*, 1981; Shaper *et al.*, 1982; Mackintosh *et al.*, 1982; DOE, 1983). The actual concentration of lead in tobacco itself is extremely variable having been reported as between 21 and 84 µg/cigarette (Franzke *et al.*, 1977). It has been estimated that the direct inhalation intake of lead from smoking 20 cigarettes a day would lie between 1 and 5 µg (WHO, 1977).

Pottery or Earthenware Glazes

Lead-glazed pottery has been known to result in lead poisoning from antiquity. The Greeks used such vessels for cooking but under carefully controlled conditions and the taboos they introduced in this respect were lost when transferred to the aristocratic class of the Roman civilisation. Indeed wine stored in this way was almost certainly contaminated by lead. In 1754, John Lind, knowing of the problems associated with lead solution from earthenware jugs, warned that lemon and wine juices should not be stored in them and finally Sir George Baker, found, in 1767, that uptake of lead into apple cider from the vessels from which it had been prepared and stored were the reasons for the Devonshire colic (Meiklejohn, 1954).

The problem of lead uptake from glazes is one associated not only with the glaze but also with the material stored in the vessel, the more acidic the material the greater its ability to dissolve lead from a glaze. This is, however, only true if the glaze has an improper mix of lead oxide and silica which leaves residual lead oxide unconverted into the lead silicate (Maquis, 1971). This can occur either because of incorrect proportions of lead oxide to lead silicate in the glaze prior to firing or alternatively because the vessel has not been glazed at a sufficiently high temperature. Where glazing takes place at temperatures greater than 1200°C, it is unlikely that any residual oxide will be left, all of it having been converted into lead silicates. Lead silicates are not readily dissolved in acid conditions (NAS, 1972).

Tests for Glaze Lead

Conditions used to test for lead content in glazes will determine the degree of uptake of material from the glaze. As much as the solution of distilled water will take up considerable quantities of lead acetate from a surface so also would hydrofluoric acid dissolve the best Edinburgh lead crystal. The initial techniques used to measure uptake of lead from glazes were based on leaching from the glazes over 24 hours with 4 per cent acetic acid. This is, however, extremely time consuming and since then the Food and Drugs Administration of the USA have developed simplified field testing techniques which require only 30 minutes of leaching with 4 per cent acetic acid (Krinitz, 1978). Increased temperatures will also enhance uptake of lead (Seth *et al.*, 1973).

On examination of 264 earthenware glaze surfaces, Klein *et al.* (1970) found that 50 per cent could have sufficient lead leached from them to make them unsafe for culinary use and between 10 and 25 per cent of these could have caused severe lead poisoning.

Earthenware vessels are more likely to be hazardous in these circumstances since they are fired at lower temperatures for which lead is a common constituent of the glaze because it imparts low surface tension and low viscosity over a wide temperature range which results in greater smoothness, lustre and brilliance to the glaze. When lead oxides are used, it is essential that the chemical composition of the glaze is carefully formulated to avoid persistent residues after the firing process. This is so because a number of cases of lead poisoning from such glazes have been described in recent times. Klein *et al.* (1970) described one death from this source where the offending acidic material was apple juice stored in an earthenware jug. A similar instance was found in New Zealand in 1976 (Hughes *et al.*, 1976). They found that fruit juice extracted around 20000 µg/l in 24 hours and in other studies values as high as 1300000 µg/l were found after storage of 3 days (Klein *et al.*, 1970). Numerous other examples of a similar nature can be found in the literature.

Gun shot

It might ordinarily be thought that wounds from retained bullets or shot gun pellets made of or containing lead would be associated with lead poisoning but this is not always the case. In fact delayed complications associated with gun shot wounds occur in only about 10 per cent of subjects. The process of solution of fragments of lead from such sources seems to be enhanced when the fragment is bathed in synovial fluid usually within a joint space (Dillman *et al.*, 1979) and can occur many years after the incident (*Lancet*, 1976). The actual composition of the projectile is also important. Some bullets are made of lead alloyed with antimony, others are jacketed in brass or copper which presents less lead surface for absorption. Other factors come into play too such as metabolic status of the person involved. Metabolic acidosis will clearly enhance the solution of lead and thyrotoxicosis with resultant hypermetabolic phases being shown to increase lead mobilisation of projectiles (Cagin *et al.*, 1978).

In past times the preparation of projectiles could also have been associated with overexposure to lead since it has been shown that lead suboxide particles are released during the moulding of bullets or ball for guns.

Retained projectiles are not, however, the only potential source of lead intoxication associated with gun shot. Some studies have shown that chronic lead absorption can result from extended exposure to lead from propellant in pistol ranges. Such lead arises from two sources. First, during firing bullets appear to fragment slightly usually because of imperfect alignment of barrel and chamber in pistols. Secondly, there is explosive vaporisation of the primer in the propellant. Such primers contain lead trinitro-resorcinate and lead peroxide. The concentrations of lead likely to be found in these circumstances can be extremely high, certainly in excess of safety limits for occupational exposure — 150 $\mu g/\mu m^3$ (National Institute for Occupational Safety and Health, 1972) in the range 1640-20899 $\mu g/\mu m^3$ (Landrigan *et al.*, 1975; Anderson *et al.*, 1979).

Battery Casings

It was common practice during the depression of the 1930s to use battery casings which had been discarded as a fuel source. The casings burnt with a hot flame and provided a free and much appreciated source of fuel in those times (NAS, 1972). These casings were heavily contaminated with both lead sulphate and lead oxides and presented a considerable hazard when used in the home. Numbers of cases of lead poisoning have been reported because of this (Chisolm and Barltrop, 1979; Dolcourt *et al.*, 1981). It is not clear whether these cases of poisoning occur by inhalation or ingestion but it would seem likely, since maximum temperatures were insufficient to vaporise lead, that the most probable course of intake was by ingestion of increased concentrations of lead in household dusts (NAS, 1972).

Metallic Lead

Metallic lead or alloys of lead are frequently used in domestic circumstances in everything from pewter-ware to weights for fishing lines. A single ingestion of a lump of metallic lead is unlikely to be a major hazard but repeated ingestion is likely to be dangerous. Evidence for this is found from the incidence of lead poisoning in swans on the Thames and in ducks in the USA where consumption of lead weights and shot as part of normal digestive processes caused decreased fertility in these birds, high levels of erythrocyte protoporphyrin and other evidence of lead poisoning (Rozman *et al.*, 1974; Goldman *et al.*, 1977; Finley and Dieter, 1978). As a consequence of such intoxication there is some evidence that raptors, birds of prey, feeding on poisoned prey may also become lead intoxicated (Benson *et al.*, 1974) providing further evidence of transfer of lead down the food chain. Other potential sources include lead for roofing and plumbing and the continued use of lead alloys in the construction of organ pipes and the potential hazard these present when acquired by children as toys when organs are dismantled, apart from the industrial risk when the organs are tuned. Children are also at risk when parents work in lead-producing or lead-using industries. Transfer of lead from work to the home on clothing has been documented as a major source of hazard to children. For this reason, high levels of industrial hygiene should be practised, where the possibility of such transfer exists.

Foodstuff Adulteration

Cases of lead poisoning following adulteration of food and indeed of wine go back into antiquity. Lead salts were used to sweeten sour wine. In more recent times lead chromate has been used to enhance the colour of curry powder. This was a common practice in the nineteenth century (Marshall, 1876) and caused an outbreak of poisoning as recently as 1968 (Power *et al.*, 1961). It is a relatively uncommon occurrence but was of sufficient importance in the middle of this century for the Food Standards Committee of the Ministry of Agriculture Fisheries and Food to comment upon the use of lead chromate to improve the appearance of turmeric (MAFF, 1948). Another interesting way in which food was found to be contaminated was during milling when rye flour was transported in an elevator which had been 'tinned' with lead (Oliver, 1891). Unusual foodstuffs or food additives are also of concern. Health food supplements containing bone for instance have been associated with lead poisoning (Crosby, 1977). This is hardly surprising when one considers that the bulk of lead in animals is stored in bone and that in consequence the ingestion of powdered bone as a calcium supplement, even from unexposed animals, must constitute a hazard.

13 AN OVERVIEW OF SOURCES

From all of the foregoing information it is easy to appreciate that the ready identification of specific sources of exposure in humans is not easily achieved although there is more than adequate information on general levels of lead (Table 13.1). The primary input point, geological lead is really of little importance. This is particularly so in modern industrial society where the input of lead from diet, the primary source, depends not upon the local sources of exposure but rather upon society's ability to transport foodstuffs from any point on the globe. Who in the UK has not eaten South African oranges at Christmas, New Zealand lamb or Californian grapes. This global mobility of food militates against the efficacy of localised control of lead pollution. The discontinuance of the use of lead arsenate as insecticide in USA and other measures taken by western society must be applauded, but not all countries are following this example.

The dietary input of lead is therefore of overwhelming import-ance in the economy of lead absorption in man (Figure 13.1), but is that proportion of exposure that man can control least not only because of global mobility and political non-compliance but also because the ultimate sources of lead in food and the proportionate inputs thereto are still a matter of conjecture. Geological lead and lead in plants is important but so also is the lead content of the air and deposition from this source onto diverse foodstuffs and human beings. The measures taken at present to alter the concentrations of lead in air from industrial and automobile use would appear to

Table 13.1: Environmental Lead Levels

Medium	Range of concentrations
Soil (upper layers)	50-10 000 μg/g
Dust (street)	200-20 000 μg/g
Water (fresh)	0.1-50 μg/l
Water (lead plumbing)	100-40 000 μg/l
Air (ambient)	0.2-2 μg/m^3
Air (high traffic density)	2-10 μg/m^3
Food	0.01-0.5 μg/g
Canned foods (lead solder)	0.05-7.44 μg/g
Paint	1-5 mg/cm^2

Figure 13.1: Sources of Human Lead Exposure

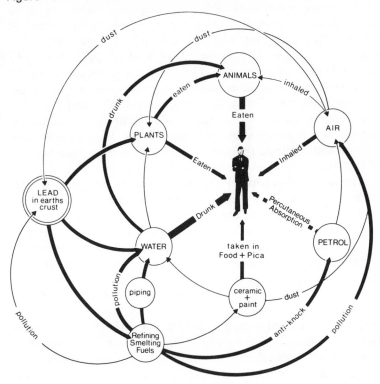

be effective. But effective only in the areas where governmental action has been taken. Large multinational oil companies continue to use as much lead alkyl as they deem necessary, especially in countries less bounded by controls exerted in Europe and USA. This type of input to the global biosphere will continue to affect populations distal to the source of exposure until it is discontinued. Discontinuance is by no means a certain guarantee of immediate decrease in exposure. The half-life of lead in the environment ensures that the global exposure to this metal will remain high probably for all time, as a consequence of the present input to the biosphere.

Control of exposure should nevertheless be attempted. The obvious controls, such as decrease and removal of lead in petrol, cessation of the use of soldered cans, removal of lead water supply systems and many many others already exist. What, however, of the so-called adventitious sources. Man in many cases is unaware of the importance of these. Who, sampling pure water acidic spring waters would suspect the hazard that lies therein? The same also for the artist, licking his brush coated with lead oxide paint. These sources are ones which can always potentially occur as 'hot' spots usually because of ignorance. Typical of this is the continued use of lead weights by the fisherman. Society today exhorts us to utilise our leisure time profitably to regenerate the mind and the body. What better sport for this than fishing? In our overcrowded society, however, so many have taken to this leisure pursuit that wildlife and particularly swans and ducks are threatened because of ingestion of lost and discarded lead weights.

The relationship between dietary, pulmonary and other sources of lead input to man depends upon a number of physical and chemical constraints. At the present time the evidence is that the dietary component is the greatest, representing at least 75 per cent of input in the normal urban environment. Pulmonary input is a lesser but significant source of exposure, whereas input through the skin may effectively be neglected. The proportions of air lead contribution to diet and dust lead contributions to air must remain a matter for investigation although more and more sophisticated experimental evidence means that we can estimate likely contributions in given situations. These situations do, however, vary widely and it is therefore unwise to try to generalise. The recommendations of the Royal Commission on Environmental Pollution and the DHSS in the UK and the National Academy of Sciences in the USA make sound sense in the light of the findings that have been presented to them. One can only hope that governments and industry will take heed and act appropriately. The quintessential nature of man's continued existence on this planet lies on his ability to control the destructive influences of colour, class, creed and environment. Only one of these colour is unchangeable others have been and can be changed. Moves to abate lead exposure lie in this category.

The conclusions of the Royal Commission on Environmental Pollution (1983) with respect to their deliberations on lead, serve well as a postscript to these chapters. They emphasise the role of food and drink, of petrol and hence air lead, the extraneous sources of paint, cans, dust, shot, fishing weights, cosmetics and finally conclude:

Our overriding concern in formulating our recommendations has been to reduce the amount of lead dispersed in the environment by man. We consider that the accumulative effect of these actions will be a substantial reduction in the rate of accumulation of lead in the environment to the benefit of present and future generations.

References to Part Two

Ali, A.R., Smales, O.R.C. and Aslam, M. (1978) Surma and lead poisoning. *Br. Med. J.*, *2*, 915-16.

Alloway, B.J. and Davies, B.E. (1971) Heavy metal content of plants growing on soils contaminated by lead mining. *J. Agr. Sci., Cambridge*, *76*, 321-3.

Anderson, K.E., Fischbein, A., Kestenbaum, D., Sassa, S., Alvares, A.P. and Kappas A. (1979) Plumbism from airborne lead in a firing range. An unusual exposure to a toxic heavy metal. *Am. J. Med.*, *63*, 306-12.

Annest, J.L. (1983) Trends in blood lead levels of the United States population. In R.R. Jones and M.J. Rutter (eds) *Lead Versus Health*. Wiley, Chichester, pp. 33-58.

Archer, F.C. (1977) Trace elements in soils in England and Wales. *Proc. ADAS Conf. Inorganic Pollution and Agriculture*. April 4-6, London.

Aslander, O. (1977) *Lead in petrol — Scope for its Reduction*. Swedish Nature Conservancy Executive.

Ault, W.U., Senechal, R.G. and Erlebach, W.E. (1970) Isotopic composition as a natural tracer of lead in the environment. *Environ. Sci. Tech.*, *4*, 305-13.

Baily, P., Kilroe-Smith, R.A. and Rendall, R.E.G. (1977) Some aspects of the biochemistry of absorption and excretion of lead and mercury, in S.S. Brown (ed.) *Clinical Chemistry and Chemical Toxicology of Metals*. Elsevier — North Holland, Amsterdam, pp. 131-6.

Beattie, A.D. Briggs, J.D., Canavan, J.S.F., Doyle, D., Mullin, P.J. and Watson, A.A. (1977) Acute lead poisoning. *Quart. J. Med.*, *XLIV*, 275-84.

—— Moore, M.R., Devenay, W.T., Miller, A.R. and Goldberg, A. (1972) Environmental lead pollution in an urban soft-water area. *Br. Med. J.*, *ii*, 491-84.

——, —— and Goldberg, A. (1972) Tetraethyl lead poisoning. *Lancet*, *ii*, 12-15.

Beattie, A.D., Mullin, P.J., Baxter, R. and Moore, M.R. (1979) Acute lead poisoning an unusual cause of hepatitis. *Scott. Med. J.*, *24*, 318-21.

Benson, W.W., Pharaoh, B. and Miller, P. (1974) Lead poisoning in a bird of prey *Bull. Env. Contam. Toxicol.*, *11*, 105-8.

Berlin, A., Amavis, R. and Langevin, M. (1977) Research on lead in drinking water in Europe (in relation to the possible uptake of lead by man). *WHO Working group on Health Hazards from Drinking Water*. London, 26-30 September.

Bertine, K.K. and Goldberg, E.D. (1971) Fossil fuel combustion and the major sedimentary cycle. *Science*, *173*, 233-5.

Betts, P.R., Astley, R. and Raine, D.N. (1973) Lead intoxication in children in Birmingham. *Br. Med. J.*, *1*, 402-6.

Billick, I.H. and Gray, V.E. (1978) *Lead Based Paint Poisoning Research. Review and Evaluation 1971-77*. HUD US Government Printing Office, Washington DC.

Bogden, J.D. and Louria, D.B. (1975) Soil contamination from lead in paint chips. *Bull. Env. Contam. Toxicol.*, *14*, 289-93.

Bose, A., Vashistha, K. and O'Loughlin, B.J. (1983) Azarcon por empacho — another cause of lead toxicity. *Paediatrics*, *72*, 106-8.

Bowen, H.J. (1975) Residence times of heavy metals in the environment, in *International Conference on Heavy Metals in the Environment.* Toronto. pp. 1-19.

Brunekreef, B., Veenstra, S.J., Biersteker, K. and Boleij, J.S.M. (1981) The Arnhem Lead Study. I Lead uptake by 1- to 3-year old children living in the vicinity of a secondary lead smelter in Arnhem, the Netherlands. *Env. Res.*, *25*, 441-8.

Bryce-Smith, D. and Stephens, R. (1981) *Lead or Health.* Conservation Society, London.

Bryan, E.H. (1974) Concentrations of lead in urban stormwater. *J. Water Poll. Control*, *74*, 2419-21.

Byers, R.K. (1959) Lead poisoning: Review of the literature and report on 45 cases, *Paediatrics*, *23*, 583-603.

Cagin, C.R., Diloy-Puray, M. and Westerman, M.P. (1978) Bullets, lead poisoning and thyrotoxicosis. *Ann. Int. Med.*, *89*, 509-11.

Campbell, B.C. and Baird, A.W. (1977) Lead poisoning in a group of demolition workers. *Br. J. Indust. Med.*, *34*, 298-304.

Carter, L. (1976) Marine pollution and sea disposal of wastes. *Chem. Ind.*, *19*, 825-9.

Center for Disease Control (1982) Blood lead levels in US population. *Morb. Mort. Weekly Report*, *31*, 132-4.

Cermak, J.E. and Thompson, R.S. (1977) Urban planning, in W.R. Boggess, (ed.) *Lead in the Environment*, National Science Foundation, Washington DC, pp. 229-39.

Chamberlain, A.C., Heard, K.J., Little, P., Newton, D., Wells, A.C. and Wiffen, R.D. (1978) *Investigations into Lead from Motor Vehicles.* Environ. Med. Sci. Div., AERE, Harwell, HMSO, London.

Chisolm, J.J. and Barltrop, D. (1979) Lead. *Arch. Dis. Child.*, *54*, 249-55.

Christison, R. (1844) On the action of water upon lead. *Trans. R. Soc. Edin.*, *15*, 265-76.

—— (1845) *Treatise on poisons* 4th edn, Black, Edinburgh, 1st edn 1829.

Craig, H., Krishriaswani, S. and Somayajulu, B.L.K. (1973) 210 Pb- 226 Ra radioactive disequilibrium in the deep sea. *Earth Planet Science Letters*, *17*, 295-305.

Crosby, W.H. (1977) Lead contaminated health food. Associated with lead poisoning and leukaemia. *J. Am. Med. Assoc.*, *237*, 2627-9.

Davies, B.E. (1971) Trace metal content of soils affects by base metal mining in the West of Scotland. *Oikos*, *22*, 366-72.

Day, J.P., Hart, M. and Robinson, M.S. (1975) Lead in urban street dust. *Nature*, *253*, 343.

De Graeve, J., Jamin, P. and Rondia, D. (1975) Plombemie d'une population adulte de l'Est de la Belgique. *Rev. Epidem. Med. Soc. et Santé Publ.*, *23*, 131-52.

DHSS (1980) *Lead and Health.* HMSO, London.

Diemel, J.A.L., Brunekreef, B., Boleij, J.S.M., Biersteker, K. and Veenstra, S.J. (1981) The Arnhem Lead Study II Indoor pollution and indoor/outdoor relationships. *Environ. Res.*, *25*, 449-56.

Dillman, R.O., Crumb, C.K. and Lidsky, M.J. (1979) Lead poisoning from a gunshot wound (Report of a case and review of the literature). *Am. J. Med.*, *66*, 509-14.

Department of the Environment (1974) *Lead in the Environment and its Significance to Man.* HMSO, London.
—— (1981) European Community screening programme for lead. United Kingdom results for 1979-1980 *Pollution Report No. 10*, HMSO, London.
—— (1982) The Glasgow Duplicate Diet Study (1979-1980) *Pollution Report No. 11*, HMSO, London.
—— (1983) European Community screening programme for lead. United Kingdom results for 1981 *Pollution Report No. 18*, HMSO, London.
Dolcourt, J.L., Finch, C., Coleman, G.D., Klimas, A.J. and Millar, C.R. (1981) Hazard of lead exposure in the home from recycled automobile storage batteries. *Paediatrics, 68*, 225-30.
Duggan, M.J. (1983) Lead in dust as a source of children's body lead, in M. Rutter and R.R. Jones (eds) *Lead Versus Health*, Wiley, Chichester, pp. 115-39.
Eastwell, H.D. (1983) Skeletal lead burden in Aborigine petrol sniffers. *Lancet, 2*, 524-5.
EEC (1975a) Council directive relating to quality of water for human consumption. *Official J. Eur. Commun., 18*, 2-17.
—— (1975b) Proposal for a council directive on air quality standards for lead. *Official J. Eur. Commun., 18*, 29-32.
—— (1976) Directive on the approximation of the laws on the member states relating to cosmetic products. *Official J. Eur. Commun., 19*, 169-200.
—— (1977) Council directive on biological screening of the population for lead. *Official J. Eur. Commun., 20*, 10-17.
Eisinger, J. (1977) Lead and man. *TIBS, 2*, 147-50.
Elias, R., Hirao, Y. and Patterson, C. (1975) Impact of present levels of aerosol Pb concentrations on both natural ecosystems and humans. *Proc. Int. Conf. Heavy Metals in the Environment, Toronto*, pp. 257-71.
Environmental Protection Agency (1976) *National Interim Primary Drinking Water Regulations.* EPA, 570/9, 76-003, Washington DC.
—— (1979) *Environmental information* EPA, 104/8, Washington DC.
Facchetti, S., Geiss, F., Gaglione, P., Colombo, A., Garibaldi, G., Spallanzani, G. and Gilli, G. (1982) *Isotopic Lead Experiment.* Commission of the European Communities, Luxembourg.
Farmer, J.G. and Lyon, T.D.B. (1977) Lead in Glasgow street dirt and soil. *The Science of the Total Environment, 8*, 89-93.
Farquar, R.M. and Fletcher, I.R. (1980) Lead isotope identification of sources of galena from some prehistoric indian sites in Ontario, Canada. *Science, 207*, 640-3.
FDA (1980) Lead acetate: Listing as a color additive in cosmetics that color the hair on the scalp. Food and Drug Administration. *Federal Register, 45*, 72112-8.
Finley, M.T. and Dieter, M.P. (1978) Influence of laying on lead accumulation in bone of mallard ducks. *J. Toxicol. Environ. Health, 4*, 123-9.
Flanagan, F.J. (1973) Values for international geochemical reference samples. *Geochem. Cosmochim. Acta, 37*, 1189-200.
Franzke, Cl., Ruick, G. and Schmidt, M. (1977) Untersuchungen zum schwermetallgehalt von tabakwaren und tabakrauch. *Die Nahrung, 21*, 417-18.
Gage, J.C. and Litchfield, M.H. (1969) The migration of lead from paint films in the rat gastrointestinal tract. *J. Oil Col. Chem. Assoc., 52*, 236-43.
Gibson, J.L., Love, W., Hardie, B., Bancroft, P. and Turner, A.J. (1892) Notes on lead poisoning as observed among children in Brisbane. *Proceedings of International Medical Congress of Australia*, 3rd Session, p. 76.
Gilfillan, S.C. (1965) Lead poisoning and the fall of Rome. *J. Occup. Med., 7*, 53-60.

Goldberg, A. and Beattie, A.D. (1972) Studies in environmental lead pollution. *Health Bull., 30,* 181-3.

Goldberg, E.D., Brocker, W.S. Gross, M.G. and Turekian, K.K. (1971) Marine chemistry, in *Radioactivity in the Marine Environment,* National Academy of Sciences, Washington DC, pp. 137-46.

Goldman, M., Dillon, R.D. and Wilson, R.M. (1977) Thyroid function in Pekin ducklings as a consequence of erosion of ingested lead shot. *Toxicol. Appl. Pharmacol., 40,* 241-6.

Graham, J.A.G., Maxton, D.G. and Twort, C.H.C. (1981) Painter's palsy: a difficult case of lead poisoning. *Lancet, 2,* 1159-60.

Grandjean, P. (1983) Health significance of organolead compounds, in M. Rutter and R.R. Jones (eds) *Lead versus Health.* Wiley, Chichester, pp. 179-89.

—— Olsen, N.B. and Hollnagel, H. (1981) Influence of smoking and alcohol consumption on blood lead levels. *Int. Arch. Occup. Environ. Health, 48,* 391-7.

Grandstaff, D.E. and Myer, G.H. (1979) Lead contamination of urban snow. *Arch. Environ. Health, 33,* 222-3.

Green, S.D.R., Lealman, G.T., Aslam, M. and Davies, S.S. (1979) Surma and blood lead concentrations. *Public Health, London, 93,* 371-6.

Hankin, L., Heichel, G.H. and Botsford, R.A. (1973) Lead poisoning from colored printing inks — a risk for magazine chewers. *Clin. paediair., 12,* 654-5.

——, —— and —— (1974a) Lead on wrappers of speciality foods as a potential hazard for children. *Clin. Paediatr., 13,* 12.

——, —— and —— (1974b) Lead content of printed polyethylene food bags. *Bull. Environ. Contam. Toxicol., 12,* 645-8.

——, —— and —— (1976) Lead on painted handles of kitchen utensils. *Clin. Paediatr., 15,* 635-6.

Harrison, R.M. (1976) Organic lead in street dusts. *J. Environ. Sci. Health, A11,* 417-23.

—— (1979) Toxic metals in street dusts and household dusts. *Sci. Total Environ., 11,* 89-97.

—— and Laxen, D.P.H. (1980) Physiochemical speciation of lead in drinking water. *Nature, 286,* 791-3.

—— and —— (1981) *Lead Pollution. Causes and Control.* Chapman and Hall, London.

Hassall, A.H. (1876) *Food. Its Adulteration and Methods for its Detection.* Longmans Green, London.

Hedley, G. and Lockley, J.C. (1975) Quality of water discharged from an urban motorway. *Water Pollution Control, 74,* 659-74.

Heichel, G.H., Hankin, L. and Botsford, R.A. (1974) Lead in paper: A potential source of food contamination. *J. Milk and Food Tech., 37,* 499-503.

Heusgem, C. and De Graeve, J. (1972) Importance de l'apport alimentaire en plumb dans l'est de la Belgique, in *Proceedings International Symposium, Environmental Health Aspects of Lead,* Amsterdam, Commission of the European Communities, Luxembourg, pp. 85-91.

Hirschler, D.A., Gilbert, L.F., Lamb, F.W. and Niebylski, L.M. (1957) Particulate lead compounds in automobile exhaust gas. *Ind. Eng. Chem., 49,* 1131-42.

HMSO (1977) Lead in drinking water. A survey in Great Britain 1975-1976. Report of an interdepartmental working group. *Pollution Paper No. 12,* HMSO, London.

Holt, L.E. (1923) Lead poisoning in infancy. *Am. J. Dis. Child., 23,* 229-33.

Hughes, J.T., Horan, J.J. and Powles, C.P. (1976) Lead poisoning caused by glazed pottery: Case report. *New Zealand Med. J., 84,* 266-8.

Hunt, W.F., Pinkerton, C., McNulty, O. and Creason, J.P. (1971) A study in trace element pollution of air in 77 midwestern cities, in *Trace Substances in Environmental Health IV*, D.D. Hemphill (ed.) Columbia University of Missouri Press, pp. 56-68.

Jaulmes, P., Hamelle, G. and Roques, J. (1960) Le plomb dans les mouts et les vins. *Ann. Tech. Agric., 9*, 189-245.

Jelinek, C.F. (1982) Lead levels in the Unites States food supply. *J. Assoc. Anal. Chem., 65*, 942-6.

Joselow, M.M. and Bogden, J.D. (1977) Lead content of printed media (Warning: spitballs may be hazardous to your health). *Am. J. Public Health, 64*, 238-40.

Karalekas, P.C., Ryan, C.R., Larson, C.D. and Taylor, F.B. (1977) *Alternative Methods for Controlling the Corrosion of Lead Pipe.* Presented at the Annual Conference of the New England Water Words Association, Boston, Massachusetts, Sept 13th.

Kato, K. (1932) Lead meningitis in infants. *Am. J. Dis. Child., 44*, 569-91.

Kjerschow, E. (1979) *Occupational Exposure to Tetra-alkyl Lead.* BSc Thesis, Env. Eng. University of Strathclyde, Glasgow.

Klein, M., Namer, R., Harpur, E. and Corbin, R. (1970) Earthenware containers as a source of fatal lead poisoning. Case study and public health considerations. *N. Engl. J. Med., 283*, 669-72.

Krinitz, B. (1978) Rapid screening field test for detecting cadmium and lead extracted from glazed ceramic dinnerware: collaborative study. *J. Assoc. Anal. Chem., 61*, 1124-9.

Lacey, R.F., Moore, M.R. and Richards, W.N. (1983) Lead in water, infant diet and blood. The Glasgow Duplicate Diet Study *Arch. Environ. Health*, in press.

Lancet Editorial (1976) Delayed lead poisoning. *Lancet, ii*, 1126.

Landrigan, P.J., Baker, E.L., Himmelstein, J.S., Stein, G.F., Weddig, J.P. and Straub, W.E. (1982) Exposure to lead from the mystic river ridge: The dilemma of deleading. *N. Engl. J. Med., 306*, 673-6.

—— McKinney, A.S., Hopkins, L.C., Rhodes, W.W., Price, W.A. and Cox, D.H. (1975) Chronic lead absorption. Result of poor ventilation in an indoor pistol range. *J. Am. Med. Assoc., 234*, 394-7.

Laug, E.P. and Kunze, F.M. (1948) The penetration of lead through the skin. *J. Industr. Hyg., 30*, 256-8.

Law, W.R. and Nelson, E.R. (1968) Gasoline sniffing by an adult. Report of a case with the unusual complication of lead encephalopathy. *J. Am. Med. Assoc., 204*, 1002-4.

Leland, H.V. and McNurney, J.M. (1974) Lead transport in a river ecosystem. *Proceedings International Conference on Transport of Persistent Chemicals in Aquatic Ecosystems.* Ottowa, pp. 17-23.

Lightfoot, J., Blair, H.J. and Cohen, J.R. (1977) Lead intoxication in an adult caused by Chinese herbal medication. *J. Am. Med. Assoc., 238*, 1539.

Lind, J. (1754) Letter to the author on the danger of using certain earthen vessels. *Scots Magazine, 16*, 227-9.

Lin-Fu, J.S. (1980) Lead poisoning and undue lead exposure in children: history and current status, in H.L. Needleman (ed.) *Low Level Lead Exposure*, Raven Press, New York, pp. 5-16.

Lockwood, J.P., Bateman, P.C. and Sullivan, J.S. (1972) Mineral resource evaluation of the US Forest Service Sierra. Demonstration project area Sierra National Forest, California. *US GS Professional Paper, 714*, Washington DC.

Lyon, T.D.B. and Lenihan, J.M.A. (1977) Corrosion in solder jointed copper tubes resulting in lead contamination of drinking water. *Br. Corr. J., 12*, 40-5.

McCord, C.P. (1953) Lead and lead poisoning in early America: The pewter era. *Ind. Med. Surg., 22*, 573-7.

McFarren, E.F., Buelow, R.W. Thurnau, R.C., Gardels, S.R., Kent, S.P. and

Dressman, R.C. (1977) Water quality deterioration in the distribution system, in *Proceedings of Water Quality Technology Conference*, Kansas City, Cincinnati.

McIntosh, M.J., Moore, M.R., Goldberg, A., Fell, G.S., Cunningham, C. and Halls, D.J. (1982) Studies of lead and cadmium exposure in Glasgow, UK. *Ecol. Dis.*, *1*, 177-84.

Maclean, A.J., Halstead, R.L. and Finn, B.J. (1969) Extractability of added lead in soils and its concentration in plants. *Can. J. Soil Sci.*, *49*, 327-34.

Ministry of Agriculture, Fisheries and Food (1948) *Food Standards Committee Report on Curry Powder*. HMSO, London.

— (1972) *Survey of Lead in Food*. Working Party on the Monitoring of Foodstuffs for heavy metals. Second report. HMSO, London.

— (1975) *Survey of Lead in Food*. Working Party on the Monitoring of Foodstuffs for heavy metals. Fifth report. HMSO, London.

— (1983) *Food Additives and Contaminants Committee Report on the Review of Metals in Canned Foods*. HMSO, London.

Maquis, J.E. (1971) Lead in glazes. Benefits and safety precautions. *Bull. Am. Ceramic Soc.*, *50*, 921-3.

Marletta, P., Favretto Gabrielli, L. and Favretto, L. (1973) Lead in grapes exposed to automobile exhaust gases. *J. Sci. Fd. Agric.*, *24*, 249-52.

Marzulli, F.N., Watlington, P.M. and Maibach, H.I. (1978) Exploratory skin penetration findings relating to the use of lead acetate hair dyes. *Curr. Prob. Dermatol.*, *7*, 196-204.

Meiklejohn, A. (1954) The mill reek and Devonshire colic. *Br. J. Ind. Med.*, *11*, 40-4.

Moore, M.R. (1973) Plumbosolvency of waters. *Nature*, *243*, 222-3.

— (1977) Lead in drinking water in soft water areas — health hazards. *Sci. Total Environ.*, *7*, 109-15.

— (1983) Lead exposure and water plumbosolvency, in M. Rutter and R.R. Jones, (eds) in *Lead versus Health*, Wiley, Chichester, pp. 79-106.

—, Goldberg, A., Fyfe, W.M. and Richards, W.N. (1981) Maternal lead levels after alteration to water supply. *Lancet*, *2*, 203-4.

—, —, Pocock, S.J., Meredith, P.A., Stewart, I.M., MacAnespie, H., Lees, R. and Low, R.A.L. (1982) Some studies of maternal and infant lead exposure in Glasgow. *Scott. Med. J.*, *27*, 113-23.

—, Hughes, M.A. and Goldberg, D.J. (1979) Lead absorption in man from dietary sources. *Int. Arch. Occup. Environ. Health*, *44*, 81-90.

—, Meredith, P.A., Campbell, B.C., Goldberg, A. and Pocock, S.J. (1977) Contribution of lead in drinking water to blood lead. *Lancet*, *ii*, 661-2.

—, —, Watson, W.A., Sumner, D.J., Taylor, M.K. and Goldberg, A. (1980) The percutaneous absorption of lead 203 in humans from cosmetic preparations containing lead acetate, as assessed by whole-body counting and other techniques. *Fd. Cosmet. Toxicol.*, *18*, 399-405.

Mcore, P.J., Pridmore, S.A. and Gill, G.F. (1976) Total blood lead levels in petrol vendors. *Med. J. Aust.*, *1*, 438-40.

Motto, H.L., Daines, R.H., Chilko, D.M. and Motto, C.K. (1970) Lead in soils and plants: Its relationship to traffic volume and proximity to highways. *Environ. Sci. Tech.*, *4*, 231-8.

Mroz, E.J. and Zoller, W.H. (1975) Composition of atmospheric particulate matter from the eruption of Heimaey, Iceland. *Science*, *190*, 461-4.

Murozumi, M., Chow, T.J. and Patterson, C. (1969) Chemical concentrations of pollutant lead aerosols terrestrial dusts and sea salts in Greenland and Antarctic snow strata. *Geochim. Cosmochim. Acta*, *33*, 1247-94.

Nagy, L., Posta, J. and Papp, L. (1976) Uber den bleigehalt in den ungarischen weinen. *Z. Levensm. Unters-Forsch, 160*, 141-2.

National Academy of Sciences (1972) *Airborne Lead in Perspective.* Washington DC.

—— (1980) *Lead in the Human Environment.* Washington DC.

National Institute for Occupational Safety and Health (1972) *Criteria for a Recommended Standard — Occupational Exposure to Lead.* Washington DC.

Nriagu, J.O. (1978) *The Biogeochemistry of Lead in the Environment.* Elsevier/North Holland, Amsterdam.

—— (1979) Global inventory of natural and anthropogenic emmissions of trace metals in the atmosphere. *Nature, 279*, 409-11.

—— (1980) Lead in the atmosophere and its effect on lead in humans. in R.L. Singhal and J.A. Thomas (eds) *Lead Toxicity* Urban and Schwartzenberg, Baltimore, pp. 483-503.

O'Brien, B.J., Smith, S. and Coleman, D.O. (1980) *Lead Pollution of the Global Environment.* Monitoring and Assessment Research Centre, Technical Report, 16.

O'Brien, J.E. (1976) Lead in Boston water, its cause and prevention. *J. N. Engl. Water Assoc., 90*, 173-80.

Ohi, G., Seki, H., Akiyama, K. and Yagyu, H. (1974) The pigeon, a sensor of lead pollution. *Bull. Environ. Contamin. Toxicol., 12*, 92-8.

Ohi, G., Seki, H., Minowa, K. Ohsawa, M., Mizoguchi, I. and Sugimori, F. (1981) Lead pollution in Tokyo — the pigeon reflects its amelioration. *Environ. Res., 26*, 125-9.

Oliver, T. (1891) *Lead Poisoning in its Acute and Chronic Forms.* Young J. Pentland, Edinburgh and London.

Packham, R.F. (1971) The leaching of toxic stabilisers for unplasticised PVC water pipe P1 and P2. *Water Treatment Exam., 20*, 108-66.

Pagenkopf, G.K. and Neuman, D.R. (1974) Lead concentrations in native trout. *Bull. Environ. Contam. Toxicol., 12*, 70-5.

Patterson, C.C. (1965) Contaminated and natural lead environments of man. *Arch. Environ. Health, 11*, 344-63.

Patterson, M. and Jernigan, W.C.T. (1969) Lead intoxication from moonshine. *GP, 40*, 127.

Pearl, K.N. (1977) Lead hazard in Asian eye cosmetic. *Lancet, i*, 315.

Porteous, J.M. (1876) *God's Treasure — House in Scotland.* Simpkin Marshall and Co, London.

Power, J.G.P., Barnes, R.M., Nash, W.N.C. and Robinson, J.D. (1961) Lead poisoning in Gurkha soldiers in Hong Kong. *Br. Med. J., 3*, 336-7.

Rastogi, S.C. and Clausen, J. (1976) Absorption of lead through the skin. *Toxicology, 6*, 371-6.

Ray, S. (1978) Bioaccumulation of lead in atlantic salmon. *Bull. Environ. Contam. Toxicol., 19*, 631-6.

Reece, R.M., Reed, J., Scott Clark, C., Angoff, R., Casey, K.R., Challop, R.S. and McCabe, E.A. (1972) Elevated blood lead levels and the in situ analysis of wall paint by x-ray fluorescence. *Am. J. Dis. Child., 124*, 500-2.

Reed, C.D. and Tolley, J. (1973) Drinking water plumbosolvency. *Lancet, i*, 1131.

Richards, W.N., Britton, A. and Cochrane, A. (1979) Reducing plumbosolvency — the effect of added lime on the Loch Katrine water supply to Glasgow. *J. Inst. Water Eng. Sci., 34*, 315-33.

—— and Moore, M.R. (1982) Plumbosolvency in Scotland. The problem, remedial action taken and health benefits observed. in *Proceedings Annual Conference American Water Works Association,* Miami, pp. 901-18.

Rieke, F.E. (1969) Lead intoxication in shipbuilding and shipscrapping 1941 to 1968. *Arch. Environ. Health, 19*, 521-39.

Robinson, J. (1981) Lead in Greenland snow. *Ecotoxicol. Environ. Safety, 5*, 24-37.

Royal Commission on Environmental Pollution (1983) 9th report — *Lead in the Environment.* HMSO, London.

Rozman, R.S., Locke, L.N. and McClure, S.F. (1974) Enzyme changes in Mallard ducks fed iron or lead shot. *Avian Diseases, 18,* 435-45.

Seth, T.D., Sircar, S. and Hasan, M.Z. (1973) Studies on lead extraction from glazed pottery under different conditions. *Bull. Environ. Contam. Toxicol., 10,* 51-5.

Settle, D.M. and Patterson, C.C. (1980) Lead in Albacore — Guide to lead pollutions in Americans. *Science, 207,* 1167-76.

Shaper, A.G., Pocock, S.J., Walker, M., Wale, C.J., Clayton, B., Delves, H.T., and Hinks, L. (1982) Effects of alcohol and smoking on blood lead in middle-aged British men. *Br. Med. J., 284,* 299-302.

Shea, K.P. (1973) Canned milk. *Environment, 15,* 6-11.

Sheldon, R.P., Warner, M.A., Thompson, M.E. and Pierce, H.W. (1953) Stratigraphic sections of the phosphuria formation in Idaho 1949. *US Geol. Survey Cric, 304,* 1.

Sherlock, J., Smart, G., Forbes, G.I., Moore, M.R., Patterson, W.J., Richards, W.N. and Wilson, T.S. (1982) Assessment of lead intakes and dose-response for a population in Ayr exposed to a plumbosolvent water supply. *Hum. Toxicol., 1,* 115-22.

Silverberg, B.A., Wong, P.T.S. and Chau, Y.K. (1976) Ultrastructural examination of *Aeromonas* cultured in the presence of organic lead. *Appl. Environ. Microbiol., 32,* 723-5.

Singer, C. and Underwood, E.A. (1962) *A Short History of Medicine,* 2nd ed, Oxford, p. 101.

Sinn, W. (1980) Uber den zusammenkang von luftibleikonzentration und bleigehalt des blutes von autohnern und berufstatgen in kerngebiet einer grosstadt. *Int. Arch. Occup. Environ. Health, 47,* 93-118.

—— (1981) Relationship between lead concentration in the air and blood lead levels of people living and working in the centre of a city (Frankfurt blood lead study). II Correlations and conclusions. *Int. Arch. Occup. Environ. Health, 48,* 1-23.

Smart, G.A., Warrington, M. and Evans, W.H. (1981) The contribution of lead in water to dietary lead intakes. *J. Sci. Fd. Agr., 32,* 129-33.

Snodgrass, G.J.A.I., Ziderman, D.A., Gulati, V. and Richards, J. (1973) Cosmetic plumbism *Br. Med. J., 4,* 230.

Stegavik, K. (1975) An investigation of heavy metal contamination of drinking water in the city of Trondheim, Norway. *Bull. Environ. Contam. Toxicol., 14,* 57-60.

Struempler, A.W. (1976) Trace metals in rain and snow during 1973 at Chadron Nabraska. *Atmos. Environ., 10,* 33-7.

Swaine, D.J. and Mitchell, R.L. (1960) Trace element distribution in soil profiles. *J. Soil Sci., 11,* 347-68.

Taylor, S.R. (1964) Abundance of chemical elements in the continental crust. A new table. *Geochim. Cosmochim. Acta, 28,* 1273-85.

Taylor, W., Molyneux, M.K.B. and Blackadder, E.S. (1974) Lead over-absorption in a population of oxy-gas burners. *Nature, 247,* 53-4.

Ter Haar, G.L. (1970) Air as a source of lead in edible crops. *Environ. Sci. Technol., 4,* 226-9.

Tola, S. and Nordman, C.H. (1977) Smoking and blood lead concentration in lead-exposed workers and an unexposed population. *Environ. Res., 13,* 250-5.

Turekian, K.K. (1977) The fate of metals in the oceans. *Geochim. Cosmochim.*

Acta., *41*, 1139-44.

—— and Wedepohl, K.H. (1961) Distribution of the elements in some major units of the earths crust. *Geol. Soc. Am. Bull.*, *72*, 175-91.

US Geological Society (1976) *Lead in the Environment.* Professional Paper No. 957, Washington DC.

Vighi, M. (1981) Lead uptake and release in an experimental trophic chain. *J. Ecotoxcol. Environ. Safety*, *5*, 177-93.

Vinogradov, A.P. (1956) Average contents of chemical elements in the earths crust. *Geochemistry*, 1-43.

—— (1962) Average contents of chemical elements in the principal types of igneous rocks of the earths crust. *Geochemistry*, 641-64.

Vives, J.F., Bellet, H., Lapinski, H., Mirouze D., Richard, J.L., Hirsch, J.L., Soulayrac, M., Mathieu-Daude, P., Vallat, G. and Michel, H. (1980) Alcoolisme chronique et intoxicationo saturnine. *Gastroenterol. Clin. Biol.*, *4*, 119-22.

Volobuev, M.I. and Golovnya, S.V. (1972) Molybdenum mercury lead and uranium content of granitic rocks of the Ensisei Range. *Vestn. Mosk. Univ. Geol.*, *27*, 66-71.

Waldron, H.A. and Stofen, D. (1974) *Subclinical Lead Poisoning.* Academic Press, London.

Ward, N.I., Reeves, R.D. and Brooks, R.R. (1975) Lead in soil and vegetation along a New Zealand State Highway with low traffic volume. *Env. Pollut.*, *9*, 243-57.

Wedepohl, K.H. (1971) Zinc and lead in common sedimentary rocks. *Econ. Geol.*, *66*, 240-2.

Wesolowski, J.J., Flessel, C.P., Twiss, S., Stanley, R.L., Knight, M.W., Coleman, G.C. and De Garmo, T.E. (1979) The identification and elmination of a potential lead hazard in an urban park. *Arch. Environ. Health*, *34*, 413-18.

Weston, R.S. (1920) Lead poisoning by water and its prevention. *N. Engl. Water Works Assoc.*, *34*, 239-63.

Wigle, D.T. and Charlebois, E.J. (1978) Electric kettle as a source of human lead exposure. *Arch. Environ. Health*, *33*, 72-8.

Wilcox, H.B. and Caffey, J.P. (1926) Lead poisoning in nursing infants. Report of two cases due to the use of lead nipple shields. *J. Am. Med. Assoc.*, *86*m, 1514-16.

Wilfon, J. (1754) An account of the disease called mill-reck. *Scots Magazine, 16*, 287-8.

Wong, C.S. and Berrang, P. (1976) Contamination of tap water by lead pipe and solder. *Bull. Environ. Contam. Toxicol.*, *15*, 530-4.

Wong, P.T.S., Chau, Y.K. and Luxon, (1975) Methylation of lead in the environment. *Nature, 253*, 263-4.

World Health Organization (1973) *The Hazards to Health and Ecological Effects of Persistent Substances in the Environment.* Report of Working Group, Stockholm.

—— (1977) *Environmental Health Criteria 3 Lead* WHO, Geneva.

—— (1982) Limit of 50 µg/l Pb *ICP/RCE 209*, (2), *279K*, 47-53.

Zielhuis, R.L., Struik, E.J., Herber, R.G.M., Salle, H.J.A., Verbek, M.M., Posma, F.D. and Jager, J.H. (1977) Smoking habits and levels of lead and cadmium in blood in urban women. *Int. Arch. Occup. Environ. Health*, *39*, 53-8.

Zimdahl, R.L. and Skogerboe, R.K. (1979) Behaviour of lead in soils. *Environ. Sci. Technol.*, *11*, 1202-8.

PART THREE

THE EFFECTS OF LEAD

-

14 METHODOLOGICAL AND STATISTICAL ISSUES

William Yule

Science is often not so much about answering questions, but about asking them — more precisely, it is about posing questions in such a way that choices can be made among possible alternative answers. From previous chapters, it is evident that 'Lead and its compounds are potentially toxic; the element has no known physiological functions; it is widely distributed in nature and, as a result, of man's activities. The gross effects which it can have on health have been recognised for many years ...' (DHSS, 1980). The problem posed to the DHSS Working Party on Lead in the Environment seemed very simple. As lead is a neurotoxin which, in large amounts, causes brain damage in children, is it likely that much lower levels of lead exposure also affect children's functioning and development, albeit in a much subtler way? Like many simple, readily understood questions, it is easy to pose but much more difficult to answer.

This chapter examines studies which have investigated the association between ordinary levels of lead exposure and children's psychological development. There have been several recent detailed reviews of the published literature up to about 1979 (Rutter, 1980; DHSS, 1980; Needleman, 1980; Needleman and Landrigan, 1981) as a result of which a number of methodological problems have been identified. Before discussing these, let us consider whether there is a question to answer in the first place.

Clarifying the Question

Seventy years ago, Thomas and Blackfan (1914) reported that lead is a neurotoxin (i.e. that it interferes with the working of the central nervous system) and that lead poisoning in children can cause encephalopathy (a syndrome characterised by gross ataxia, repeated vomiting, lethargy, stupor, convulsions, headaches, hallucinations, tremor and coma. See Winneke, Chapter 15).

Some children survive an acute encephalopathy but are often left with a variety of permanent neurological and psychological

193

impairments (Smith *et al.*, 1963; Smith, 1964; Perlstein and Attala, 1966). Clearly, large doses of lead are dangerous. But how can one find out whether lower doses might also have adverse effects on health and development?

The most powerful way of investigating such a question is to carry out controlled experiments. For obvious, ethical reasons, such experiments cannot be carried out on children. Investigators have to rely on less powerful, indirect methods of enquiry. For example, it is generally more acceptable to carry out experimental studies on animals and results of such studies are discussed in more detail in Chapter 15. For present purposes, it is sufficient to note that by giving lead in the diet of nursing rats, similar encephalopathies are produced in the animals as were found in children who had been accidentally poisoned (Pentschew and Garro, 1966). Studies of the effects of lead on rats have to be conducted very carefully as there is an interaction between high leaded diets and consequent poor nutrition (Mahaffey and Michaelson, 1980). Because of this, it is not clear whether any change in the rats' behaviour is caused directly by the ingestion of lead or by the distorted diet. Where diet has been properly controlled, the evidence shows that even relatively small traces of lead can interfere with a wide variety of physiological, biochemical and neurochemical functions, most noticeably in neuronal systems utilising acetylcholine, catecholamines and gamma-aminobutyric acid (GABA) as neurotransmitters (Silbergeld and Hruska, 1980; Silbergeld, 1983).

In other words, the results of carefully controlled animal studies show that small traces of lead interfere with the normal working of the central nervous system. Silbergeld and Hruska (1980) conclude that '... neurochemical studies caution against assuming the existence of a "safe" level of lead exposure and raise concerns that the neuron may be irreversibly damaged by any exposure to lead.' More recent work in Germany has shown that increased lead levels in primates interfere with their ability to learn new skills (Lilienthal *et al.*, 1983). Thus, there is strong evidence that there is a case to answer.

In the face of this evidence, it is a reasonable hypothesis that low level lead exposure may have adverse effects. But it is still an hypothesis. The fact that there is a case to answer does not mean that it has been proven that low levels of lead do cause damage to children. To take it further, it is necessary to ask whether there are human studies which are compatible with the hypothesis that lead at low doses has harmful effects.

In adults, it has been found that lead levels as low as 10 to 20 μg/100 ml inhibit the haem biosynthetic pathway. This raises the worry that there could be a lowering of the amount of oxygen available in the central nervous system (Bridbord, 1980). Studies of adult lead workers find that the rate at which messages are passed along peripheral nerves is slowed down. This slowing of nerve conduction velocity was evident across the whole range of blood lead levels (Araki and Honma, 1976). There is, therefore, some evidence both of biochemical effects of lead at low dosages and of a relationship with nerve conduction velocities — both of which are concordant with a 'no-threshold' hypothesis.

Recently, two sets of studies have looked at children's EEGs (their electroencephalographic records which indicates the activity of the brain) and both studies claim that relatively low lead exposures are associated with measurable EEG differences. Burchfiel *et al.* (1980) compared the EEGs of 22 children with 'low' lead and 19 with 'high' lead selected from the groups examined in detail by Needleman *et al.* (1979) (see below). The authors reported that the high lead children showed more slow waves which are characteristic of younger or developmentally delayed children.

Potentially, this way of examining children is very important because it is looking for changes at a neurophysiological level and such measures are less likely to be affected by confounding social factors (see below) than are psychological measures. However, this particular set of results has to be treated with caution as the number of children involved was small, the sample was highly selected, it is not really clear what the EEG measures mean, and since the authors studied 320 EEG variables, some of the apparently positive studies could have occurred by chance.

The second set of studies was conducted with children aged 13 to 75 months who had blood leads in the normal range (Benignus *et al.*, 1981; Otto *et al.*, 1981, 1983). They recorded EEGs while the children were involved in a sensory conditioning task. They found that the amount of slow wave voltage varied as a linear function of blood lead level. There was no evidence of any threshold operating, and so their results provided evidence of altered CNS function at very low lead levels.

Again, one has to be cautious in interpreting these results

because the EEG measures have not been used previously and no one is really sure what they mean. However, whatever they mean, there is evidence that changes occur and are related to body lead burden.

Taken all together, evidence from these studies is compatible with the hypothesis that low levels of lead exposure are associated with changes in CNS functioning. Moreover, there is no evidence for the existence of some threshold below which lead has no effect. But being compatible with an hypothesis and proving a case are two different things.

Evidence from Early Studies

In 1943, Byers and Lord described a study of 20 children who had been admitted to hospital, mainly before the age of 2 years, because of lead intoxication. Most of the lead got into the children's body because they put all sorts of things into their mouths and ate them — often described as 'pica', after the magpie (Latin name, *Pica pica*) who takes anything. The majority of the affected children came from deprived backgrounds. When the children were reassessed during their primary school days, only one child was making satisfactory progress. As a group, they showed a high frequency of educational and behavioural problems. Byers and Lord focused attention on the possibility that lead intoxication played some part in interfering with normal psychological development.

This classic study not only drew attention to the potential hazard to children's development, it also illustrates the major methodological problem facing research in this area. Educational and behavioural problems are known, even more clearly now than in 1943, to be associated with deprived social backgrounds. How can the social influences be separated from any independent influences of the action of lead? Indeed, does lead have any direct, independent action on children or is it merely an indirect index of social circumstances? The problem has been posed for a quarter of a century. How nearer are we to a solution?

Methodological Considerations

There is now considerable agreement among researchers in the field as to the major methodological problems which have to be considered by each research study. Seven methodological considerations have been identified in recent reviews (Needleman *et al.*, 1979; Rutter, 1980; Ernhart, Landa and Schell, 1981 a and b; Needleman and Landrigan, 1981; Cowan and Leviton, 1980).

1. Assessment of Body Lead Burden

The amount of lead in a child's body at any one point in time can only be estimated by one of a number of different measurements. Some measures are more difficult to take than others, and an estimate of how much lead is currently in the child's body may be a poor indicator of the level of lead to which that child has been exposed in the past.

The measurement techniques for blood lead levels are well established and can have good reliability (US Environmental Protection Agency, 1977; Vahter *et al.*, 1982; WHO, 1984). It is important that the blood sample is obtained properly, as it is all too easy for the blood sample to be contaminated. This is why it is preferable to get blood from a vein rather than by pricking the finger. If the finger is dirty, any trace of lead in the dirt will greatly distort the estimate of the lead in the child's blood.

To emphasise the care with which samples have to be taken, consider the following. In Britain today, the average blood lead level of high risk school children is in the region of 15 µg/100 ml (DHSS, 1980; DOE, 1981, 1983). A concentration of 10 µg/100 ml can be expressed as 4 parts per million (ppm). Trying to identify one part per million is like trying to identify one second out of a three week time period — such are the levels of traces of lead we are interested in identifying. Thus, if the sample is allowed to get dirty, the results could easily be wrong.

Once the sample is taken to a laboratory, the lead content is measured by a process called atomic absorption spectography. This is an elaborate and sophisticated technique and it requires great care to ensure that different laboratories can produce similar estimations (Vahter, 1982). In a well-organised laboratory, the amount of error of measurement can be reduced to about 2 µg/100 ml. That is, if a sample is estimated to contain 10 µg/100 ml, then the chances are 67 in 100 that a second reading from the same sample will lie in the range 8-12 µg/100 ml, and 95 in 100 that the true reading lies in the range 6-14 µg/100 ml. Notice that here we are talking of the accuracy of the measurement, not the fluctuations in the child's body lead burden.

Most studies have relied on a single estimation of lead in blood. It is widely accepted that one estimate of blood lead gives an indication of the amount of lead circulating in the blood at only one point in time and may be a poor index both of overall body lead burden and of long-term exposure to lead (DHSS, 1980; Cowan and Leviton, 1980). Even so, blood lead is one of the most reliable indices of recent lead exposure, particularly in relation to environmental sources (DHSS, 1980). Provided the environmental exposure has remained the same, blood lead can give some indication of exposure over time. In one of the few studies to examine the question (Otto *et al.*, 1982), it was found that blood lead estimates taken two years apart showed reasonable stability ($r = +0.64$).

Thus, where one is interested in long-term exposure to presumed constant sources of lead pollution, then a single estimate of blood lead level may well be a useful index. However, it will not distinguish between children who have had acute episodes of higher lead levels and those who have not. The body does get rid of most of the lead ingested from diet, water and air so that *current* body lead burden tells us little about past exposure. A raised blood lead level is a reasonable index of recent or current high exposure, but a normal level does not rule out previous chronic or acute lead exposure.

Many of the problems of using blood lead as a marker of total body lead burden could be overcome by the use of repeated blood lead levels over a lengthy time span. Unfortunately, taking venous blood samples from children is a potentially unpleasant experience, and it is unclear whether it is ethically justifiable to use such invasive procedures with children who are not individually at risk of some clinical problem. What other methods are there?

Radiological measurement of the deposition of lead in the long bones provides a better indication of chronic, high level lead exposure. However, X-rays are not sufficiently sensitive to identify lower levels of lead exposure, and by their very nature are intrusive and dangerous. A variety of biochemical markers is possible, but some are so specialised as not to be generally available for large-scale research studies, while others involve the administration of chelation agents which have their own risks attached (Chisholm, 1965; Cowan and Leviton, 1980).

In the late 1970s, a new marker of body lead burden was developed — the analysis of the lead content of teeth. Lead is stored in all bones, and is laid down in teeth over considerable time periods, with little getting lost by normal chelation processes. Thus, by collecting children's teeth as they were shed, it became possible to get an index of cumulated lead exposure.

Tooth lead estimates show moderate agreement with blood lead estimates (De la Burdé and Choate, 1972; Needleman and Shapiro, 1974; De la Burdé and Shapiro, 1975; Needleman *et al.*, 1979). Unfortunately, there are major variations in the estimates of tooth lead level according to the precise way in which the tooth is analysed, dentine having a different uptake of lead than enamel, for example. Different teeth may absorb lead at different rates (Delves *et al.*, 1982) and even in the same child, estimations from two different teeth can result in contradictory findings (Needleman *et al.*, 1979). Laboratory standards are not as well developed for the estimation of tooth lead as for blood lead. Another factor which has to be borne in mind is that one has to wait for the teeth to be shed naturally. This occurs usually between the ages of 5 and 8 years — an inconveniently early age for undertaking psychological assessments, particularly of academic attainment. Moreover, during any one time period, some children will not lose any teeth so that these children cannot be included in a study. Since there is some evidence that brighter children are more likely to donate teeth (Smith *et al.*, 1983), this adds new biases to cross-sectional studies.

The situation regarding the estimation of body lead burden has been well summarised by Rutter (1980):

It is evident that no single approach is entirely satisfactory. Probably serial blood levels constitute the best measure, but they are only infrequently practicable. Dentine lead is likely to prove the next best alternative, provided the technical problems can be mastered. Single blood lead levels have the great merit that we know a great deal about their meaning, but the major defect that they provide no guide to the *duration* of current exposure or to the existence of *past* exposure. All these considerations mean that the differentiation of high-lead and low-lead exposure groups (especially on single blood estimations) will be somewhat unreliable, therefore the differences in outcome between them are likely to constitute an *underestimate* of the true differences between populations with chronically increased and with acceptably low levels of lead exposure.

2. Assessment of Children's Behaviour and Intelligence

Without a clear model of the effects of lead on children, it is difficult to select appropriate measures which will be sensitive to low level lead exposure. In the absence of models from animal studies or from other sources, investigators have resorted to using broad measures of general intelligence together with a potpourri of less well-validated measures, supposedly sensitive to neurological dysfunction.

It is widely agreed that tests administered simultaneously to groups of children can be used as *screening* instruments in large-scale studies, but are insufficiently sensitive to pick up the sorts of deficits in intelligence, attention and so on that might be expected. The most widely used and best validated individual test of cognitive functioning — the Wechsler Intelligence Scale for Children — Revized (WISC-R) (Wechsler, 1974) — taps a wide range of intellectual functioning. However, it is costly both in skilled manpower and time to administer.

The WISC-R yields three estimates of intelligence — Verbal Intelligence (based on 5 subtests), Performance Intelligence (based on a different 5 subtests) and Full Scale IQ (based on all ten subtests). These measures are known to be reliable. Individual subtests, being very much shorter, have considerably more error of measurement and are less reliable. Despite years of use as a research and clinical tool, there are considerable limits to the inferences one can make from WISC scores about CNS functioning (Rutter *et al.*, 1970; Chadwick and Rutter, 1983). The WISC-R is sensitive to severe head injury but is less sensitive to milder injuries resulting in post-traumatic amnesia of less than three weeks (Chadwick *et al.*, 1981a and b). If even the WISC-R is not sensitive to known head injury, how far can one expect it to be sensitive to lesser degrees of cerebral dysfunction?

It is now widely accepted that it does not make sense to talk of 'brain damage' in children as if it were a global entity. Rather, it is increasingly recognised that damage to or dysfunction in localised areas of the brain will be associated with particular losses of functioning. The quest for the perfect test of 'brain damage' has been largely abandoned (Herbert, 1964), but people still try to infer brain damage from the pattern of scores on general tests such as the WISC-R. Even though the evidence for this is very weak (Rutter *et al.*, 1970a), these old concepts have influenced the strategy for trying to identify CNS deficits in children exposed to lead. The argument is that if lead is a neurotoxin, then it should have greater effects on Performance IQ than on Verbal IQ. As has just been argued, the evidence for Verbal-Performance discrepancies as indices of brain damage is weak, and as will be seen in later chapters, if anything, children with higher lead levels do worse on verbal tests than on non-verbal ones.

The validity of other measures of neuropsychological functioning is even less agreed (Chadwick and Rutter, 1983). The validity of even such widely used test batteries as the Halstead-Reitan battery (Reitan, 1974) is still a matter of considerable controversy (Boll, 1981; Boll and Barth, 1981). Different investigators have tried to measure different functions, and all of these variations in methodology make it difficult to draw conclusions from apparently contradictory findings.

Recently, there has been renewed interest in obtaining psycho-physiological measures which are presumed to reflect CNS functioning fairly directly and to be largely independent of learning and social influences. Reaction time has been measured by a number of investigators (Landrigan *et al.*, 1975; Needleman *et al.*, 1979). Unfortunately, they have tended to use a variety of different reaction time procedures and give little rationale for the particular paradigm chosen (Ernhart, *et al.*, 1981b). The same criticism applies to measures of finger tapping. Some investigators have used EEG measures (Burchfiel *et al.*, 1980; Benignus *et al.*, 1981; Otto *et al.*, 1981, 1983), but they have used novel indices whose validity has not been established.

Many investigators comment on disturbances of attention in children with higher lead levels. Indeed, disturbances of attention are commonly implicated in a variety of learning difficulties. Despite this, there is little consensus in the developmental neuro-psychological literature on how best to assess different aspects of attention (Taylor, 1980). Some authors have inferred attentional difficulties from scores on reaction time tasks (Needleman *et al.*, 1979), and others have used a continuous performance task. In this, the child has to watch a continually changing display of, say, letters of the alphabet and has to press a button when an X is shown. Variations on this task are used by different investigators, and again, its validity as a measure of attention is not clearly established (Chadwick *et al.*, 1981c).

From this, it is clear that research into the presumed effects of lead on children's neurological functioning is hampered in a number of ways. First, there are no widely agreed models of what lead may do to the CNS or how this will be manifested in behaviour. Secondly, although tests of general intelligence and of scholastic attainment are well standardised, are reliable, and give valid measures, the results of such tests cannot be easily used to infer subtle changes in functioning. Thirdly, the validity of most of the experimental tests of CNS functioning has not been adequately established. Fourthly, different forms of experimental procedures are used so that it is difficult to compare results from different studies. Given the comparatively small number of studies that have been published, it is little wonder that it is difficult to come to firm conclusions about the effect of lead on children's development.

The situation regarding the measurement of children's *behaviour* is marginally better. Parents, teachers, other adults and even children themselves can be asked to report on whether or not they show a particular piece of behaviour. Such measures have what is called 'face' validity in so far as they look as if they are really measuring what they say they are measuring. However, there are problems.

Behaviour is usually measured by asking someone whether a particular description applies to a particular child. The parent may be asked to say whether Johnnie is 'restless', and if so whether such a description of his behaviour 'certainly applies' or only 'applies somewhat'. In other words, the adult is asked to rate the applicability of the description on a three point scale. It is left up to the adult to make the finer-grained distinction and clearly, this will depend on a host of factors such as how many children the adult is familiar with, on how well they know the particular child, and even on how well they like the child. There are opportunities for all sorts of bias to creep in. Obtaining good ratings of behaviour requires much more than simply putting a whole lot of descriptions together to form a questionnaire. The better scales have been tried and tested on many thousands of people so that ambiguities in wording are removed and the sort of scores likely to be obtained in particular subgroups of children are established. Two sets of measures which have been carefully developed and well standardised are the Conners Teachers' Questionnaire (Conners, 1969) and the Parents and Teachers Behaviour Rating Scales developed by Rutter (Rutter, 1967; Rutter *et al.*, 1970a). The former was developed to focus on hyperactive behaviour and has been shown to be sensitive to changes in children's behaviour following drug treatment. The latter cover a wider spectrum of behaviour and have been shown to be very good screening instruments for use with large groups of children.

One complicating factor in assessing children's behaviour is the well-established but awkward fact that children behave very differently at home and at school (Mitchell and Shepherd, 1966; Rutter *et al.*, 1970b). It is not uncommon for children who are overactive at home to be very quiet and well-behaved at school, and vice versa. A recent study has found that the few children who are overactive in both settings differ qualitatively from those who are overactive in only one of the situations (Schachar *et al.*, 1981). Thus, it is advisable to get information on children's behaviour from both home and school, and to get it on a wide spectrum of behaviours.

Once again, until clearer hypotheses are formulated to relate lead level to behaviour, it is probably necessary to continue to use relatively large batteries of tests and scales covering a wide range of functions. The better standardised the instruments, the more likely are clear results to be noted. However, all psychological tests can be sensitive to testers' biases, so it is essential that examiners remain 'blind' to the body lead burden of the children they are testing or rating until after the data are scored.

3. Problems with Test Batteries

The more tests that are included in a test battery, the greater the likelihood that some of the observed differences, say between high and low lead groups, will arise merely by chance. When a study reports that a particular difference between two groups is statistically significant, with a probability of $P < 0.05$, this means that there are fewer than 5 chances in 100 that the difference could have arisen by chance. Put another way, if a battery of twenty tests has been given, one would expect that, on average, one of the tests would show a 'significant' difference at the 0.05 level by chance alone.

Where the tests in a battery are intercorrelated, as is the case with most batteries used in lead research, then the probability of observing a chance difference rises markedly. Ernhart *et al.*, (1981b) calculated that since Needleman *et al.*, (1979) measured

52 different variables, the probability of obtaining one or more differences which is statistically significant at the $P = 0.05$ level by chance is 0.93 and not 0.05 as is commonly believed. Each dependent variable (outcome measure) should not be considered separately. Instead, some form of multivariate analysis should be performed on the data set.

The two most satisfactory guides as to whether any differences are merely chance fluctuations are: (1) whether the significant differences always fall in the same direction. Where one is dealing with chance fluctuations, they should favour each group equally. Thus, on some measures the high lead group would appear to perform better than the low lead group, and vice versa on other measures; (2) whether the same differences arise in different investigations. Chance factors should not produce the same pattern of findings in different studies. Ultimately, *replication*, and not the application of statistics, is the best test of whether a finding is meaningful and can be generalised to other samples.

4. Sample Size and Levels of Statistical Significance

Whether a difference between two groups reaches statistical significance depends on factors such as the size of the difference, the variability within samples, and the size of the samples studied. It is quite possible for a real, but small, difference between two populations to appear to be *not* statistically significant when only small samples are studied. Likewise, trivial differences between two samples may be statistically significant if the two samples are sufficiently large.

When experimenters conclude that there is a statistically significant difference in the average scores of two defined groups, they are saying that there is a greater variability *between* the groups than there is *within* the groups. For example, if one was interested in whether circus dwarfs were less tall than policemen, it would be easy to see that when the heights of the individuals were plotted on a graph that all the dwarfs' heights clustered around, say, 4ft 6in whereas the policemen's heights clustered around 5ft 11in and *the two distributions of scores did not overlap.* Clearly, (and not surprisingly) there is a significant difference in the average heights of the two groups. Statistics are not necessary to reflect the obvious, but in the more usual problems facing experimenters, the distributions of scores (say on IQ tests) overlap between the contrasting groups (say of high and low lead exposed children). Various statistical techniques of analysis of variance can be used to test whether, despite the overlapping distribution of scores, the two groups can reasonably be regarded as separate. The greater variability in scores within each group, and the greater the overlap of the distributions, then the less likely it is that any apparent difference reflects a true difference. This is illustrated in Figure 14.1. Alas, for research in the lead field, there is considerable variability in IQ scores at all levels of lead exposure and it is difficult to reach clear-cut answers.

No amount of statistical argument can help in deciding whether a particular difference between two groups is clinically meaningful. Rather, the investigators have to use their knowledge about a particular test to judge whether the observed difference is in accordance with what they know. Ideally, they should have some model of the action of lead which they use to predict the magnitude of differences on any one test. For example, children of professional parents regularly score some 10 to 20 points higher than children of unskilled workers on tests of general intelligence. These are large differences, and yet a range of 20 points — from 90 to 110 — encompasses 50 per cent of the population. Given that these social class differences are clearly established, one has to hazard a guess as to whether the differences between high and low lead groups will be of this order of magnitude, even greater or very much less. Most investigators would probably guess that the expected difference would be less than 10 points. Given this expectation, it is possible to estimate in advance the size of samples necessary to investigate hypotheses accurately (Cowan and Leviton, 1980; Schlesselman, 1974; Freiman *et al.*, 1978). Where other factors are going to be investigated and controlled statistically, even larger samples of children will be required.

5. Biased Ascertainment of Subjects

The purpose of undertaking small studies is to draw firm conclusions that can be applied to the total population. If the children studied are not representative of the total population, then the results of the study may be specific to the groups tested. Ideally, samples should be drawn at random from populations, but this cannot always be done. Rather, investigators take advantage of the availability of groups of children whose lead levels are known, and

Figure 14.1: Possible Distributions of IQ Scores of Low and High Blood Lead Groups. In all three cases, there is the same average IQ for each of the lead groups, but the small scatter of scores in (a) makes it likely the two groups really differ in terms of IQ whereas in (c) the overlap between the distributions makes it less likely

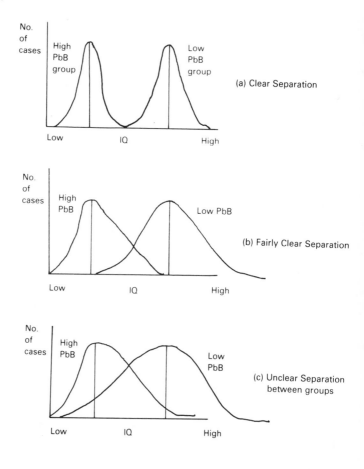

then describe the group in terms of social class and other demographic characteristics to judge how like the total population they are.

However, it is widely accepted that where highly selected groups of children are studied, unknown biases may radically affect the results. To take an example from another field. There was a long controversy concerning the relative importance of neurological and emotional problems in the aetiology of reading disability. Not surprisingly, investigators who worked in neurological clinics got different results from those based in child guidance clinics. It is easy to see, now, that they were probably investigating different types of children. Only epidemiological studies — studies based on sampling total populations — can help avoid such biases (Rutter and Yule, 1975; Cowan and Leviton, 1980).

Even population studies have their problems. It is impracticable to test all children, so samples are drawn. Not everyone sampled wants to participate, some families cannot be traced, some may be rejected by the investigators on a variety of grounds. Unless these grounds are specified beforehand, it is difficult to avoid the suspicion of biased rejection. Voluntary drop-outs do not occur at random. It is well established in epidemiological studies that those subjects who do not participate are at higher risk of having deviant characteristics (Cox *et al.*, 1977). Indeed, a recent large scale study of tooth lead levels found that bright girls were more likely to donate teeth than less bright boys, thereby producing a hitherto unsuspected source of bias (Smith *et al.*, 1983).

6. Threshold Effects

There is considerable controversy over whether lead has a cumulative effect which begins at minute levels of exposure, or whether there is one or more thresholds beyond which impairment can be assessed. Many studies have compared a 'high' and a 'low' lead group, but this strategy is very limiting since it cannot reveal anything about the nature of the relationship between lead and dependent variables. Without any idea of what happens in the middle, one cannot infer the form of any dose-response relationship.

Where extreme groups have been compared, too often the cut off levels have been decided arbitrarily, and it is impossible to pool data from different studies. It must also be noted that what one study labels as 'low' may be regarded as 'high' in another study. Very few studies before 1980 looked at really low levels and most were comparing 'high' lead with even 'higher' lead exposure.

7. Cause, Consequence or Correlate? The Problem of Confounding Variables

Cross-sectional research studies — which constitute the bulk of the studies examining the relationship between lead and children's development — are bedevilled by the need to distinguish between correlation and causation. Many studies report *associations* between exposure to lead and a variety of indices of development, but does the association represent a cause or a consequence of lead exposure or are both the raised lead levels and the cognitive/ behavioural deficits due to the operation of some third set of factors. This is a very real problem, not just a theoretical nicety. Lead is not randomly distributed throughout the population. Children who live in disadvantaged circumstances are exposed to more lead, and this shows in large differences in blood lead levels between socioeconomic groups. The US NHANES II survey (Annest *et al.*, 1982) demonstrates that urban children have higher mean blood levels than rural children; children who live in families with low incomes have higher blood lead levels than those with high incomes; and irrespective of income or place of residence, black children have much higher lead levels than white children. All these factors — place of residence, social deprivation and race — are related to children's performance on tests of intelligence and attainment. How can one determine what proportion of the variation in IQ, say, is due to lead, how much to social factors, and how much to a combination of the two.

Or take the example of pica. The eating of inedible substances is more frequent in less intelligent and more behaviourally disturbed children (Bicknell, 1975), and in turn, pica exposes children to lead. In this case, the relationship can operate in both directions simultaneously — behavioural disturbance increases exposure to lead which results in more behavioural disturbance. In other words, pica can be both a symptom of behavioural disturbance and a cause of it through lead intoxication.

The whole problem of inferring the causal nature of an association from correlation data is extremely complex, but vital to our understanding. Two examples will serve to illustrate the difficulties. The first, unconnected with lead, is quoted by Clegg (1982). She notes that there is a very high (strong) correlation between the lengths of peoples' right and left arms. Knowing this, no one would conclude that the length of the right arm determined (caused) the length of the left arm. Rather, most people would see that the two variables do not interact at all but are '... both determined by other factors such as genetic make-up or diet, which affected both arms equally' (Clegg, 1982, p. 134). This underlines the point that a strong correlation indicates some sort of connection between the variables, but the connection need not be a direct one.

The second example comes from a dispute over the interpretation of data from the NHANES-II study (Annest, 1983; Royal Commission on Environmental Pollution, 1983). As summarised earlier in Figure 6.13 it can be seen that over the period 1976 to 1980 the average blood lead level of people in the USA dropped by 37 per cent on average from 15.8 µg/100 ml to 10.0 µg/100 ml. During this same period, the total amount of lead used in petrol in the USA declined in parallel. Indeed, the correlation was +0.95 — almost as high as possible. Since the average intake of lead through diet *increased* marginally over this five year period, changes in eating habits could not account for the lowering blood lead levels. Many environmentalists hailed the correlational data as clear proof that a reduction of lead in petrol had directly caused a reduction in blood lead levels.

While this may be one plausible explanation of the data, as noted in the right-left arm correlation example, the deduction of causality from correlation is not logically simple. Needless to say, the petroleum companies strongly contested the simple causal explanation and produced other data to suggest alternative explanations. However, the efforts of the petroleum industry to reanalyse the NHANES-II data have been severely criticised (Rosenblatt *et al.*, 1983; Annest *et al.*, 1983; Pirkle, 1983). The independent statistical review concluded that the drop in blood lead levels over the five years was a true fall, and not an artefact of measurement or sampling factors, and that there was a strong correlation between petrol-lead usage and blood lead levels. They examined the assumptions made by the various groups of statisticians and concluded that the petroleum industry '... analyses contribute little to understanding the association between blood lead and gasoline lead because the variables adopted to represent lead exposure are deemed inappropriate' (Rosenblatt *et al.*, 1983).

Attempting to unravel the complex set of interactions has important scientific and social policy implications. Until we fully understand the extent, nature and directions of the relationship among body lead burden, children's development and social factors, we will not be in a position to take the most effective action to protect our children. Without such fuller understanding, inappropriate action might be taken.

For example, if the relationship between lead level and IQ is an artefact — that is, lead level is a crude index of social factors and it is poor stimulation in the home rather than lead which is associated with lower IQ — then reducing the level of lead in the environment will make no appreciable differences to children's intelligence. In that case, it would be better to concentrate efforts in other social measures. Note that we are *not* saying that the association is an artefact, merely pointing out the implication if it were.

If it appears that there is a real association, then a different set of problems has to be considered. Does the relationship hold across all children, or are some groups — poorer, inner-city, black, younger, poorly nourished — more vulnerable than others? If there are high risk groups, these need to be identified. If biologically all children are equally vulnerable but certain environmental factors — of diet or social stimulation — *protect* some children, it would be important to identify such protective mechanisms. The interactions between body lead burden, social factors and children's development are complicated and call for sophisticated methodologies to investigate them (Rutter, 1983).

Fortunately, causality can be inferred from correlation data by following a few ground rules. First, if the association between lead and IQ persists after a wide range of background variables are taken into account statistically, then a causal connection is more likely. Secondly, a causal connection is more believable if there is a consistent linear 'dose-response' relationship between increasing lead level and some dependent index of development. Thirdly, the argument for a causal relationship is strengthened if *changes* in lead exposure or in lead levels are followed by changes in the children's behaviour or cognitive performance. The experimental method in which one factor is systematically altered while the other, independent factor is observed is the most powerful way of establishing a causal connection. Clearly, it is unethical to do this with lead and children — hence the need for indirect methods.

Bradford Hill (1977) elaborated these ground rules which are widely followed in medical epidemiological studies. However, his rules have to be modified to apply to psychological morbidity data rather than medical mortality data. For example, Hill argues that causality is more likely where the *association is strong*. This is so in the case of inferring a causal link between smoking and lung cancer, but it cannot apply when considering lead intake and intelligence test scores since we know that the variation in IQ scores is determined by a multiplicity of factors — genetic, biological and social. It is unlikely that exposure to any one heavy metal is likely to make much difference compared with the effects of nutrition or early social stimulation. If low level lead exposure had been a major determinant of IQ, it is likely that the effect would have emerged despite the many methodological problems of earlier studies. Instead, it is more believable that if lead and IQ are causally related, then only a modest proportion of variance in IQ will be shared with lead. Hill's ground rule should be amended to include reference to the expected strength of the association based on an understanding of the nature of the variables concerned.

Causality is more likely where there is *consistency of the observed association.* As noted earlier, replicability of results is essential. The relationship should be *biologically* (and psychologically) plausible. This chapter opened by indicating that it is biologically and psychologically plausible to entertain the hypothesis that if very high levels of lead cause serious damage, then lower levels may cause less damage. Finally, Hill asks whether the evidence as a whole is *coherent.* Until the nature of the action of lead on the human CNS is better understood, coherence can only be inferred from studies which address the question indirectly.

Given that intelligence test scores are determined by a multitude of factors, then one expects that lead and IQ will share only a limited proportion of the total variance of intelligence. Multivariate analysis of variance models and step-wise regression models allow us to estimate the *relative* contribution of lead and socioeconomic factors to intelligence. It is of little interest to find that socioeconomic status (SES) accounts for more of the variance in IQ than does lead. As has been argued here, that is to be expected. What really is of interest is to know that if lead accounts for, say, 5 per cent of the IQ variance, then what proportion of that variance is *really* due to lead and what to the indirect effects of SES.

The different methods of analysis make different assumptions about the metric properties of SES indices (Yule *et al.*, 1981). Usually, a harsh assumption (some call it a conservative assumption) is made whereby any shared variance is ignored and only residual variance accounted for by lead is interpreted. This assumes that when lead and SES share variance with IQ, the 'real' causal link is with SES and not with lead — the very hypothesis being investigated. By examining lead's contribution last in a step-wise regression analysis, for example, this conservative approach is adopted. It is a harsh test and may not reflect the real world. Once again, investigators need to be aware of the assumptions under-lying the statistical tools they employ and the limitations their analytical techniques may impose on the fuller understanding of their data.

Concluding Comments

It has been emphasised throughout this chapter that without clear models of how lead may be affecting children's central nervous systems, it is difficult to conduct definitive studies. It is important that both measures of body lead burden and of development are made using reliable, valid and replicable techniques. Appropriate research designs must be employed, taking care to ensure that as few biases as possible are introduced by either the selection or the subsequent loss of subjects. Where many tests are administered, care must be exercised in interpreting apparently significant results. Above all, it is vital to consider how best to control for social and other potentially confounding variables.

As far as children are concerned, it is unethical to consider an experimental study in which children's lead levels are manipulated. However, it is acceptable to monitor children's behaviour when their high lead levels are brought down by treatment. Given the immense difficulties in inferring causality from cross-sectional studies, a better, but far more expensive, strategy would be to follow a cohort of children longitudinally and measure their lead levels, behaviour and intelligence at a number of different points in time.

There can never be one perfect study which manages to control for all factors, but at least successive studies can avoid simple errors and each can deliberately investigate different aspects of remaining problems. Ideally, some will attempt the important task of attempting to repeat methodologies precisely. Why replication is prized in the physical sciences and undervalued in the social sciences remains a mystery. Without replication, most results can at best serve as hypotheses for further work.

References

Annest, J.L. (1983) Trends in blood lead levels in the United States population. in M. Rutter and R. Russell Jones (eds) *Lead Versus Health: Sources and Effects of Low Level Lead Exposure*. Wiley, Chichester, pp. 33-58.
—— , Mahaffey, K.R., Cox, D. and Roberts, J. (1982) Blood lead levels for persons 6 months - 74 years of age: United States 1976-80. *Advance Data, 79*, 1-23.
—— , Pirkle, J.L., Makus, D., Neese, J.W., Bayse, I.D. and Kovar, M.G. (1983) Chronological trend in blood-lead levels between 1976 and 1980. *New Engl. J. Med., 308*, 1373-7.
Araki, S. and Honma, T. (1976) Relationships between lead absorption and peripheral nerve conduction velocities in lead workers. *Scand. J. Work Environ. Health, 2*, 225-31.
Benignus, V.A., Otto, D.A., Muller, K.E. and Seiple, K.J. (1981) Effects of age and body lead burden on CNS function in young children. II. EEG spectra. *Electroenceph. Clin. Neurophysiol., 52*, 240-8.
Bicknell, D.J. (1975) *Pica: A Childhood Syndrome*. IRMMH Monograph No. 3. Butterworths, London.
Boll, T.J. (1981) The Halstead-Reitan neuropsychology battery, in S.B. Filskov and T.J. Boll (eds) *Handbook of Clinical Neuropsychology*. Wiley, New York, pp. 577-607.
—— and Barth, J.T. (1981) Neuropsychology and brain damage in children, in S.B. Filskov and T.J. Boll (eds) *Handbook of Clinical Neuropsychology*. Wiley, New York, pp. 418-52.
Bradford Hill, A. (1977) *A Short Textbook of Medical Statistics*. Hodder & Stoughton, London.
Bridbord, K. (1980) Low-level exposure to lead in the workplace, in H. Needleman (ed.) *Low Level Lead Exposure: The Clinical Implications of Current Research*. Raven Press, New York.
Burchfiel, J., Duffy, F., Bartels, P.H. and Needleman, H.L. (1980) Combined discriminating power of quantitative electroencephalography and neuropsychologic measures in evaluation of CNS checks of lead at low levels, in H. Needleman (ed.) *Low Level Lead Exposure: The Clinical Implications of Current Research*. Raven Press, New York, pp. 75-90.
Byers, R.K. and Lord, E.E. (1943) Late effects of lead poisoning on mental development. *Am. J. Dis. Child., 66*, 471-94.
Chadwick, O. and Rutter, M. (1983) Neuropsychological assessment, in M. Rutter (ed.) *Developmental Neuropsychiatry*. Guilford Press, New York.
—— , —— , Brown, G., Shaffer, D. and Traub, M. (1981b) A prospective study of children with head injuries: II cognitive sequelae. *Psychol. Med., 11*, 49-61.
—— , —— , Shaffer, D. and Shrout, P.E. (1981c) A prospective study of children with head injuries: IV. Specific cognitive deficits. *J. Clin. Neuropsychiat., 3*, 101-20.
—— , —— , Thompson, J. and Shaffer, D. (1981a) Intellectual performance and reading skills after localized head injury in childhood. *J. Child Psychol. Psychiat., 22*, 117-39.
Chisholm, J.J. (1965) Chronic lead intoxication in children. *Devel. Med. Child Neurol., 7*, 529-36.
Clegg, F. (1982) *Simple Statistics: A Course Book for the Social Sciences*. Cambridge University Press, Cambridge.
Conners, C.K. (1969) A teacher rating scale for use in drug studies with children. *Am. J. Psychiat., 126*, 884-8.
Cowan, L. and Leviton, A. (1980) Epidemiologic considerations in the study of the

sequelae of low level lead exposure. in H.L. Needleman (ed.) *Low Level Lead Exposure: The Clinical Implications of Current Research*. Raven Press, New York.

Cox, A., Rutter, M., Yule, B. and Quinton, D. (1977) Bias resulting from missing information: some epidemiological findings. *Br. J. Prev. Soc. Med., 31*, 131-6.

De la Burdé, B. and Choate, M.S. (1972) Does asymptomatic lead exposure in children have latent sequelae. *J. Pediat., 81*, 1088-91.

—— and Shapiro, I.M. (1975) Dental lead, blood level and pica in urban children. *Arch. Environ. Health, 30*, 281-4.

Delves, T., Clayton, B., Carmichael, A., Bubear, M. and Smith, M. (1982) An appraisal of the analytical significance of tooth lead measurement as possible indices of environmental exposure of children to lead. *Ann. Clin. Biochem., 19*, 329-37.

Department of the Environment (DOE) (1981) European Community screening programme for lead: United Kingdom results for 1979-1980. *Pollution Report No. 10.* DOE, London.

—— (1983) European Community screening programme for lead: United Kingdom results for 1981. *Pollution Report No. 18.* DOE, London.

Department of Health and Social Security (DHSS) (1980) *Lead and Health* The Report of a DHSS Working Party on Lead in the Environment. (Lawther Report). HMSO, London.

Ernhart, C.B., Landa, B. and Schell, N.B. (1981a) Subclinical levels of lead and developmental deficit — a multivariate follow-up reassessment. *Pediatrics, 67*, 911-19.

——, ——, —— (1981b) Lead levels and intelligence (letter). *Pediatrics, 68*, 903-5.

Freiman, J.A., Chalmers, T.C., Smith, H. and Kuebler, R.R. (1978) The importance of beta, the type II error and sample size in the design and interpretation of the randomized control trial. *N. Engl. J. Med., 299*, 690-4.

Herbert, M. (1964) The concept and testing of brain damage in children: a review. *J. Child Psychol. Psychiat., 5*, 197-216.

Landrigan, P.G., Whitworth, R.H., Balch, R.W., Staehling, M.W., Barthel, W.F. and Rosemblum, B.F. (1975) Neuropsychological dysfunction in children with chronic low-level lead absorption. *Lancet, i*, 708-12.

Lilienthal, H., Winneke, G., Brockhaus, A., Molik, B. and Schlipkoter, H-W. (1983) Learning-set formation in rhesus monkeys pre- and post-natally exposed to lead. *Heavy Metals in the Environment*: Proc. Int. Con., *Heidelberg*, September 1983. CEP Consultants, Edinburgh, pp. 901-6.

Mahaffey, K. and Michaelson, I.A. (1980) Interaction between lead and nutrition, in H.L. Needleman (ed.) *Low Level Lead Exposure: The Clinical Implications of Current Research*. Raven Press, New York.

Mitchell, S. and Shepherd, M. (1966) A comparative study of children's behaviour at home and at school. *Br. J. Educ. Psychol., 36*, 248-54.

Needleman, H.L. (ed.) (1980) *Low Level Lead Exposure: The Clinical Implications of Current Research*. Raven Press, New York.

——, Gunnoe, C., Leviton, A., Reed, M., Peresie, H., Maher, C. and Barrett, P. (1979) Deficits in psychological and classroom performance of children with elevated dentine lead levels. *N. Engl. J. Med., 300*, 689-95.

—— and Landrigan, P.J. (1981) The health effects of low level exposure to lead. *Ann. Rev. Pub. Health, 2*, 277-98.

—— and Shapiro, I.M. (1974) Dentine lead levels in asymptomatic Philadelphia school children: subclinical exposure in high and low risk groups. *Environ. Health Perspectives, 7*, 27-31.

Otto, D.A., Benignus, V.A., Muller, K.E. and Barton, C.N. (1981) Effects of age and body lead burdens on CNS function in young children. I. Slow cortical potentials. *Electroenceph. Clin. Neurophysiol.*, *52*, 229-39.

—, —, —, —, Seiple, K., Prah, J. and Schroeder, S. (1982) Effects of low to moderate lead exposure on slow cortical potentials in young children: A two year follow-up study. *Neurobehav. Toxicol. Terat.*, *4*, 733-7.

—, —, —, — (1983) Changes in CNS function at low-to-moderate blood lead levels in children, in M. Rutter and R. Russell Jones (eds.) *Lead Versus Health: Sources and Effects of Low Level Lead Exposure.* Wiley, Chichester, pp. 319-31.

Pentschew, A. and Garrow, F. (1966) Lead encephalo-myelopathy of the suckling rat and its implications for the porthrinopathic diseases. *Act. Neuropathol.*, *6*, 266-78.

Perlstein, M.A. and Attala, R. (1966) Neurologic sequelae of plumbism in children. *Clin. Pediatr.*, *5*, 292-8.

Pirkle, J.L. (1983) Chronological trends in blood lead levels in the United States between 1976 and 1980. Paper presented at International Conference on Heavy Metals in the Environment, Heidelberg, September 1983.

Reitan, R.M. (1974) Psychological effects of cerebral lesions in children of early school age, in R.M. Reitan and L.D. Davison (eds.) *Clinical Neuropsychology: Current Status and Applications.* Wiley, New York, pp. 53-84.

Rosenblatt, J.R., Smith, J., Royal, R., Little, R. and Landis, J.R. (1983) *Report of the NHANES II Time Trend Analysis Review Group, June 15, 1983.* North Carolina: US Environmental Protection Agency.

Royal Commission on Environmental Pollution (1983) *Ninth Report: Lead in the Environment.* HMSO, London.

Rutter, M. (1967) A children's behaviour questionnaire for completion by teachers: preliminary findings. *J. Child Psychol. Psychiat.*, *8*, 1-11.

— (1980) Raised lead levels and impaired cognitive/behavioural functioning: A review of the evidence. *Devel. Med. Child Neurol.*, *22*, Suppl. 42.

— (1983) Statistical and personal interactions: Facets and perspectives, in D. Magnusson, and V. Allen (eds.). *Human Development: An Interactional Perspective.* New York: Academic Press.

—, Graham, P. and Yule, W. (1970a) *A Neuropsychiatric Study in Childhood.* Clinics in Developmental Medicine 35/36. Heienmann/SIMP, London.

—, Tizard, J. and Whitmore, K. (eds.) (1970b) *Education, Health and Behaviour.* Longmans, London. (Reprinted Huntington, NY: Krieger, 1981).

— and Yule, W. (1975) The concept of specific reading retardation. *J. Child Psychol. Psychiat.*, *16*, 181-97.

Schachar, R., Rutter, M. and Smith, A. (1981) The characteristics of situationally and pervasively hyperactive children: implications for syndrome definition. *J. Child Psychol. Psychiat.*, *22*, 375-92.

Schlesselman, J.J. (1974) Sample size requirements in cohort and case-control studies of disease. *Am. J. Epidemiol.*, *99*, 381-4.

Silbergeld, E. (1983) Experimental studies of lead neurotoxicity: Implications for mechanisms, dose-response and reversibility, in M. Rutter and R. Russell Jones (eds.) *Lead Versus Health: Sources and Effects of Low Level Lead Exposure.* Wiley, Chichester.

Silbergeld, E.K. and Hruska, R.E. (1980) Neurochemical investigations in low level lead exposure, in H.L. Needleman (ed.) *Low level lead Exposure: The Clinical Implications of Current Research.* Raven Press, New York.

Smith, H.D. (1964) Pediatric lead poisoning. *Arch. Environ. Health*, *8*, 256-61.

—, Baehner, R.L., Carney, T. and Majors, W.J. (1963) The sequelae of pica with and without lead poisoning. A comparison of the sequelae five or more years later. I: clinical and laboratory investigations. *Am. J. Dis. Child.*, *105*, 609-16.

Smith, M., Delves, T., Lansdown, R., Clayton, B.E. and Graham, P. (1983) The effects of lead exposure on urban children. Institute of Child Health/University of Southampton study. *Devel. Med. Child Neurol. 25*, Suppl. 47.

Taylor, E. (1980) Development of attention, in M. Rutter (ed.) *Scientific Foundations of Developmental Psychiatry.* Heinemann Medical, London, pp. 185-97.

Thomas, H.M, and Blackfan, A.D. (1914) Recurrent meningitis, due to lead, in a child of five years. *J. Dis. Child., 8*, 377-80.

US Environmental Protection Agency (1977) *Air Quality Criteria for Lead* EPA-6CC/8-77-017. Washington, DC, US Government Printing Office.

Vahter, M. (ed.) (1982) *Assessment of Human Exposure to Lead and Cadmium Through Biological Monitoring.* Stockholm: National Swedish Institute of Environmental Medicine and Department of Environmental Hygiene, Karolinska Institute.

Wechsler, D. (1974) *Manual of the Wechsler Intelligence Scale for Children — revised.* Psychological Corporation, New York.

World Health Organization (WHO) (1984) *Studies in Epidemiology on Exposure of Elderly to Cadmium, Lead Neurotoxicity in Children, Welders' Exposures to Chromium and Nickel.* Health Aspects of Chemical Safety, Interim Document 15. Copenhagen: World Health Organization.

Yule, W., Lansdown, R., Millar, I.B. and Urbanowicz, M.A. (1981) The relationship between blood lead concentration, intelligence and attainment in a school population: a pilot study. *Devel. Med. Child Neurol., 23*, 567-76.

15 ANIMAL STUDIES

Gerhard Winneke

Need for Animal Models of Behaviour Disorder

As discussed in Chapter 16, clear-cut evidence on lead-induced psychological deficit in asymptomatic children is lacking so far; both positive and negative reports on hyperactivity and/or cognitive impairment in lead-exposed children have been given. This controversial state of affairs is not surprising because low level lead effects may well be less pronounced than those of confounding variables (Winneke *et al.*, 1983). Even if psychological deficit had convincingly been shown to be associated with elevated levels of environmental lead-exposure the question of direction of causality still remains: Does lead cause the deficit? Is a psychological deficit causative for increased lead absorption, as e.g. in cases of pica? Are psychological deficit and increased lead levels influenced by a third variable, such as social-economic background? (See Chapter 14 for a full discussion.)

Although multivariate regression techniques have been developed within epidemiology to deal with complex networks of interdependent variables, direct supporting evidence can be achieved only by animal experimentation. If such experiments are meant to provide models for psychological dysfunction in man, the methods developed in the tradition of experimental and comparative psychology would seem particularly useful to contribute to a clarification of the behavioural toxicity of lead. Behaviour as treated in experimental psychology may either be learned (conditioned) or unlearned (unconditioned). If learned, the learning principle may either be Pavlovian, namely governed by mere temporal contiguity of stimulus and response, or instrumental, namely governed by the consequences of behaviour. If unlearned, the behaviour may either be spontaneous or emitted, e.g. motor activity, or stimulus elicited (respondent), e.g. reflexive behaviour.

Behavioural outcome measures most frequently taken in animal lead studies are motor activity and different types of instrumental learning. These studies may be used to answer the following main questions: (1) Does lead cause behavioural deficit? (2) What is the no-effect-level (NOEL) in terms of blood lead levels (PbB)? (3) Are these effects persistent or reversible? These questions will be dealt with in the subsequent review using hyperactivity and learning deficit as behavioural outcome dimensions.

The Cause-Effect-Issue: Encephalopathy and Hyperactivity

A typical clinical picture of acute lead intoxication is encephalopathy, a syndrome characterised by gross ataxia, repeated vomiting, lethargy, stupor, convulsions, headache, hallucinations, tremor and coma. Approximately 25 per cent of all children surviving acute lead encephalopathy present with severe irreversible neurological and neuropsychological symptoms (Smith *et al.*, 1963; Perlstein and Attala, 1966).

Autopsy of brains of fatal cases often reveal characteristic morphological alterations, such as oedematous swelling and congestion. On microscopic examination findings of cerebral oedema, endothelia, hypertrophy and hyperplasia, as well as proliferation of perivascular glia, have been described (Blackman, 1937; Pentschew, 1965). This neuropathology is similar in adults and in children.

Early efforts to produce this neuropathology in adult rodents failed completely (Pentschew, 1958). A breakthrough towards finding an adequate animal model for lead encephalopathy occurred, however, when Pentschew and Garro (1966) produced characteristic neuropathology in suckling rats, whose lactating dams were given 4 per cent lead carbonate in the diet; their milk contained 46 ppm lead. At weaning 90 per cent the weanlings developed paraplegia of their extremities and more than 80 per cent of them died. Their neuropathology was characterised by haemorrhages, capillary damage, glial proliferation and areas of transudation, mainly in cerebellar and striatal structures. This animal model of lead encephalopathy has been confirmed by others (Goldstein *et al.*, 1974; Krigman and Hogan, 1974).

The Pentschew and Garro (1966) model of preweaning lead exposure has frequently been used in behavioural studies as well. Sauerhoff and Michaelson (1974) fed a diet containing 4 per cent lead acetate to lactating rats and continued lead exposure in the offspring with a diet containing 25 mg Pb/kg, equivalent to the lead concentration in the milk of their lead-fed dams. An increase of motor activity equivalent to 150-190 per cent of controls was observed. Treated animals exhibited reduced body weight, however, and no blood lead concentrations were measured.

Similar but even more striking activity increase was reported in mice (Silbergeld and Goldberg, 1973, 1974). According to the Pentschew and Garro (1966) model animals were initially exposed through their dams milk and subsequently through lead in drinking water (0, 2.5 and 10 mg/l). Treated animals from all exposure groups exhibited increased locomotor activity equivalent to 300-400 per cent of controls. The body weight of these animals was only 30-50 per cent of controls, however, and no blood lead concentrations were given.

The question must be raised, therefore, if lead can really be considered the primary cause of the observed hyperactivity, or if lead-related undernutrition during early developmental stages might serve as a more appropriate explanation. It has, in fact, been shown (Castellano and Oliverio, 1976) that mere undernutrition in mice during the early phases of brain development may produce marked delay of neurological development as well as hyperactivity. A review of the literature (Bornschein *et al.*, 1980) reveals, indeed, that less extreme conditions of lead exposure do not produce dramatic hyperactivity and in most cases no change of activity at all. Out of nine studies reporting increased activity levels associated with lead exposure six were associated with undernutrition as well (Bornschein *et al.*, 1980). It may, thus, be concluded that lead-related hyperactivity in animal studies, if observed at all, is most likely to be causally related to lead-induced undernutrition during the early developmental stages of brain development.

The next section will discuss the question whether the same argument holds true for lead-related cognitive impairment, as tested through behavioural paradigms of learning and memory.

The No Effect-Level (NOEL): Learning-deficit

A review of the earlier literature in this field (EPA, 1977) reveals that a large portion of work published before 1977 suffers from two major weaknesses: high levels of lead exposure as exemplified by the Pentschew and Garro (1966) paradigm, and poor documentation of tissue levels. The contribution of such studies to establish no-effect-levels (NOEL) for lead based on blood lead concentrations is only limited, therefore. Much of the work published since then has taken this criticism into consideration. The present review will be restricted to those more recent studies of learning which allow one to relate observed effects to blood lead levels. Such studies are briefly summarised in Table 15.1. They differ mainly (a) in terms of species or strains, (b) in terms of the exposure protocol, and (c) in terms of the learning-paradigm used.

The preferred species in these studies is the rat. This preference is not primarily based on toxicological considerations, but rather on the wealth of experience available for this species from comparative psychology, namely from studies on learning and memory. A few studies have used monkeys as their animal model (Bushnell and Bowman, 1979a, b; Rice and Willes, 1979; Lilienthal *et al.*, 1983), which allow for more direct extrapolation to cognitive performance in man.

Three main exposure protocols have been used: (1) the neonatal model with either indirect or direct lead exposure; (2) the postweaning model, with direct lead exposure usually starting at weaning at about postnatal age 21 days (PND 21), and extending through subsequent developmental stages until testing at adult age; (3) the prenatal-postnatal model including indirect maternal lead exposure during prenatal and preweaning stages plus postweaning direct exposure until testing.

The different behavioural paradigms used vary greatly; straightforward comparability of results is therefore difficult. A rough classification of tasks according to negative and positive reinforcing contingencies may prove helpful, however. In procedures using negative reinforcement animals have to avoid punishment (e.g. electric footshock) by taking appropriate action. Passive avoidance tasks involve training an animal to withhold a response in order to avoid being shocked. One-way active avoidance tasks require an animal to shuttle from an 'unsafe' compartment to a 'safe' one in order to escape from or avoid shock. In the two-way active avoidance task animals learn to shuttle from one compartment to another in order to avoid being shocked by making use of some type of warning signal; unlike one-way avoidance the animals have to learn to return to the compartment, where they have just been shocked.

Another approach to assess learning performance is by using positive reinforcing contingencies, such as food-reward in food-deprived animals. Mazes and similar devices have been used to test

Table 15.1: Recent Studies on Lead Effects on Animal Learning

Reference	Species	Exposure protocol	Blood lead Weaning	$(\mu g/100ml)$ Testing	Learning task	Observed effects
Angell and Weiss (1982)	rat	neonatal and/or postweaning testing at PND 58-130	—	C = 2 / Pb = 64-66	operant FI/FR	Inter-response times dalayed in Pb-groups
Bushnell and Bowman (1979a)	Monkey (*M.mulatta*)	neonatal for 12 months testing at 20-40 weeks	—	C = 5 / Pb_1 = 37 / Pb_2 = 58	WGTA discrimination-reversal	Pb-groups impaired
Bushnell and Bowman (1979b)	Monkey (*M.mulatta*)	Pb-exposure stopped at 12 months, testing at 48 months	—	C = 4 / Pb_1 = 5 / Pb_2 = 6	WGTA discrimination-reversal	Pb-groups impaired
Coryslechta and Thompson (1979)	rat	post-weaning testing at PND 55-140	—	C = 3-6 / Pb_1 = 7 / Pb_2 = 25 / Pb_3 = 43	operant FI	*response-rates:* increase in Pb_1, and Pb_2; decrease in Pb_3
Gross-Selbeck and Gross-Selbeck (1981)	rat	(1) postweaning / (2) pre- and neonatal testing at PND 180	—	(1) C = 6.2 Pb = 22.7 / (2) C = 3.7 Pb = 4.6	operant DRH	(1) tendency for higher rates in Pb-group / (2) higher rates in Pb-group
Hastings *et al.* (1977)	rat	neonatal testing at PND 90-186	C = 11 / Pb_1 = 29 / Pb_2 = 42	—	successive VDL (brightness)	none
Hastings *et al.* (1979)	rat	neonatal testing at PND 120-300	C = 11 / Pb_1 = 29 / Pb_2 = 65	—	(1) simult. VDL / (2) T-maze / (3) go/no-go	(1) Pb_2 impaired / (2) none / (3) none
Lilienthal *et al.* (1983, 1985)	Monkey (*M.mulatta*)	prenatal and postnatal testing at 30-50 months	—	C = 10 / Pb_1 = 35-51 / Pb_2 = 71-130	WGTA learning Set-Form	Pb_1 and Pb_2 impaired

Table 15.1 continued

Study	Species	Protocol			Test	Result
Milar *et al.* (1981)	rat	neonatal testing at PND 50	—	C = 5 Pb₁ = 26 Pb₂ = 123	operant spatial alternation	none

Overmann (1977)	rat	neonatal (direct) testing at PND 27, 70 and 100	C = 15
			Pb₁ = 33
			Pb₂ = 173
			Pb₃ = 226
				—	(1) avoidance
					  active
					  passive
					(2) Operant inhibition
					
					(3) E-maze
						(1) Acquisition and extinction impaired for Pb₃
						(2) Failure of inhibition in all Pb-groups
						(3) none

Petit and Alfano (1979)	rat	neonatal testing at PND 66-115	C = 2 Pb₁ = 331 Pb₂ = 1297	—	(1) Hebb-Williams (2) Passive avoidance	(1) none (2) Pb₁ and Pb₂ impaired
Rice and Willes (1979)	Monkey (*M. fascicularis*)	from birth through 1st year testing at PND 431-700	—	C = 5 Pb = 20-50	WGTA discrimination reversal	Pb-group impaired
Taylor *et al.* (1982)	rat	pre- and neonatal testing at PND 11	C = 3.7 Pb₁ = 38.2 Pb₂ = 49.9	—	runway (suckling as reward)	none for acquisition; extinction delayed in Pb-groups
Winneke *et al.* (1977)	rat	pre- and postnatal until testing at PND 100-140	C = 1.7 Pb = 26.6	— 28.5	easy VDL difficult VDL	none impairment
Winneke *et al.* (1983)	rat	as above testing at PND 100-150	—	C = 1.5 Pb = 16.8-24.9	easy VDL difficult VDL	none impairment

Notes: Abbreviations: C = control-group; Pb = lead exposure group; PND = postnatal day; DRH = differential reinforcement of high rates; FI = fixed interval-reinforcement; FR = fixed ratio-reinforcement; VDL = visual discrimination learning; WGTA = Wisconsin general test-apparatus.

if animals exhibit disruption of learning peformance after lead treatment. A frequently used procedure is discrimination learning; the type of discrimination can be spatial or sensory. Spatial discrimination may be simple T-mazes or complex sequences of T-mazes such as the Hebb-Williams maze. Visual discrimination learning (VDL) has also been used by several groups to study lead-induced impairment. More complex versions of discrimination learning, such as discrimination reversal learning or learning set formation have primarily been used in primates. Finally, operant procedures, i.e. modification of lever pressing responses within different schedules of reinforcement, have also been used in a number of studies.

In terms of outcome there is pronounced inter- and intratask variability. Spatial discrimination procedures, such as E-, T- and Hebb-Williams mazes (Overmann, 1977; Hastings *et al.*, 1979; Petit and Alfano, 1979) or operant spatial discrimination (Milar *et al.*, 1981) have generally proved insensitive to the effects of lead. More consistent findings have been reported for simultaneous visual discrimination learning (VDL) with brightness- or pattern-stimuli, as well as for different operant procedures.

As far as low-level effects are concerned four of the rat studies (Cory-Slechta and Thompson, 1979; Gross-Selbeck and Gross-Selbeck, 1981; Winneke *et al.*, 1977, 1983) as well as all of the primate studies are particularly relevant and will therefore be described in more detail.

Learning Disorder at Low PbB: Rat Studies

Cory-Slechta and Thompson (1979) gave lead as lead acetate in drinking water (25, 150 and 500 mg Pb/l) to Sprague-Dawley rats from weaning at PND 20-22 to testing at PND 55-60. This gave rise to average blood lead values (PbB) of about 7, 25 and 43 µg/100 ml, as compared to control levels of about 3-6 µg/100 ml (read from a graph on page 153 of this paper). The behavioural paradigm was an operant fixed interval schedule of reinforcement (FI-30), i.e. a food pellet was given at the first bar-press after at least 30 seconds delay following the last reinforcement. As compared to control level, peak response rates were about +250 per cent for the 25 and 150 mg lead groups, but about −50 per cent for the high lead group; the same tendency was observed for response latencies, i.e. shorter ones for both low level groups and longer ones for the 500 mg group. Although, in terms of PbB, these findings are less convincing for the 25 mg group, the results are generally compatible with a NOEL of PbB below 30 µg/100 ml.

Another study of this group (Cory-Slechta *et al.*, 1981) has not been listed in Table 15.1, because only brain lead levels without reference to PbB were given. This study does, however, support the conclusion drawn above: response-duration was shorter in both lead groups (50 and 150 mg Pb/l) as compared to controls, with measures taken in a bar pressing task requiring a specified duration of bar depression before pellet delivery.

Gross-Selbeck and Gross-Selbeck (1981) used two different exposure protocols in Wistar rats: direct post weaning dietary lead exposure (500 mg Pb/kg diet; as lead acetate) until testing at PND 180, and indirect maternal exposure during prenatal and pre-weaning development only. This gave rise to average PbB of 22.7 µg/100 ml in the postweaning group at PND 180, and of 20.5 µg/100 ml in lead-treated dams at weaning. PbB of controls and of maternally exposed animals at PND 110 was between 3 and 6 µg/100 ml. Using 'Differential Reinforcement of High Rates (DRH)' as the operant procedure lead-treated animals exhibited higher bar-pressing rates than controls; this effect was more pronounced only in maternally exposed animals as compared to those from the postweaning exposure group. This study, thus, supports a NOEL around 20 µg/100 ml and is generally in keeping with the behavioural findings of Cory-Slechta and Thompson (1979) and Cory-Slechta *et al.* (1981).

Interesting within-task variability of outcome is illustrated by the studies of Winneke *et al.*, (1977, 1983) in Wistar rats. Dietary lead (750 mg and 250 mg/kg diet, respectively) was given indirectly from conception until weaning and continued directly afterwards until testing between about PND 100-190. Resulting PbB from the 750 mg/kg diet was 26.6 µg/100 ml at weaning and 28.5 µg/100 ml at testing (Winneke *et al.*, 1977), and between 16.8 and 24.9 µg/100 ml at testing between PND 100-150 from the 250 mg Pb/kg diet (Winneke *et al.*, 1983); PbB of controls was below 5 µg/100 ml in both studies. Simultaneous, non-spatial visual discrimination learning (VDL) for stripe patterns differing in orientation (easy task) and for disc patterns differing in diameter (difficult task) were used to assess learning performance. The main results from both studies in terms of errors/day are given in Figure 15.1. Whereas error decrease with days of training is steep for the

Figure 15.1: Average Learning-Curves from Visual Discrimination Learning (VDL) in Rats, Taken from Different Experiments. (a) Results from an experiment with pre- and postnatal dietary lead exposure (250 mg Pb/kg diet); (b) results from an earlier study in which higher lead concentrations were given (750 mg Pb/kg diet) according to the same exposure-protocol. Each point is an average across ten animals. The abscissa represents days of training, the ordinate percentage errors per day of training

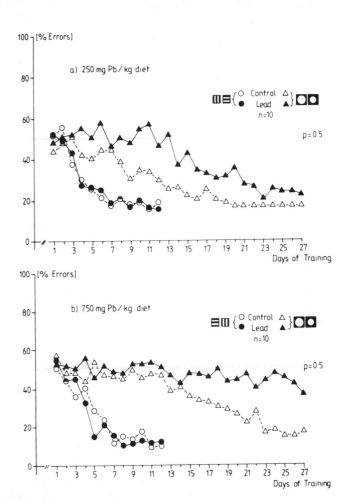

Source: (a) Winneke *et al.* (1983); (b) Winneke *et al.* (1977)

easy stripe pattern, it is much smoother for the disc pattern. In both experiments there is no exposure-related impairment for the easy stripe pattern, whereas in both instances rate of learning is retarded in lead-exposed animals for the difficult disc pattern. These effects occurred in the absence of signs of overt toxicity, as for example reduced litter size or weight or weight-loss. Since the lowest effective PbB in these studies was about 17 μg/100 ml, a NOEL below 20 μg/100 ml is compatible with these findings.

Another study from this group may be used to strengthen this conclusion (Winneke *et al.*, 1982). This study was not listed in Table 15.1 because, instead of giving PbB values directly, these were inferred from systematic feeding studies (Schlipkoeter and Winneke, 1980), and validated by measuring inhibition of erythrocyte aminolaevulinic acid dehydratase activity (ALA-D). The same exposure protocol as described above was used. VDL performance for the difficult disc pattern only was assessed in animals having received lead as lead acetate (250 and 750 mg/kg diet) until testing between PND 190-250. PbB for these exposure conditions was estimated at 18 and 31 μg/100 ml, respectively, which corresponds to the measured values given above. In addition to VDL performance two-way active avoidance learning was measured in a different set of same treated animals between PND 70-100. Whereas, as before, significant impairment of VDL performance without pronounced dose-effect gradation occurred for both groups of lead-exposed animals, significant dose-dependent improvement of active avoidance learning was observed. This unexpected finding which is, however, consistent with earlier findings from Driscoll and Stegner (1976), demonstrates that, depending on the demand characteristics of the learning task, lead-induced alterations of normal neuronal functioning may either be disruptive, as in difficult VDL tasks, or adaptive, as in shock-motivated avoidance tasks.

Learning-Disorder at Low PbB: Primate-Studies

The four primate studies listed in Table 15.1 used rhesus monkeys as experimental subjects, and the Wisconsin General Test Apparatus (WGTA) as the apparatus. Bushnell and Bowman (1979a) fed lead acetate dissolved in milk to newborn rhesus monkeys so as to achieve PbB levels of about 50 (low; n=4) and 80 μg/100 ml (high; n=4), as compared to control animals (n=4) with PbB around 5 µg/100 ml. Lead exposure started at birth and was terminated at twelve months of age. In a series of four experiments discrimination reversal learning was tested between 20 and 40 weeks of age. The animals were first trained to criterion on a two-stimulus discrimination. Afterwards the reinforcement contingencies were reserved and the animals were retrained to criterion. Although no group differences were observed for original learning, both lead groups exhibited retarded reversal learning. In terms of the NOEL discussion it should be noted that for low level- animals PbBs varied between 30 and 50 µg/100 ml. In subsequent experiments it was shown that the observed deficit was unrelated to lead-induced changes in motivation.

In a second study from this group (Bushnell and Bowman, 1979b) discrimination reversal learning was repeated well after discontinuation of Pb exposure at normalised blood lead levels. The results from this study bear on the reversibility issue and will, therefore, be discussed below.

In using a discrimination reversal paradigm Rice and Willes (1979) made an effort to replicate the findings of Bushnell and Bowman. Four controls (PbB 5 µg/100 ml) and four lead-treated monkeys (20-50 µg/100 ml), who received lead as lead acetate in milk solution from PND 1 through the first year of life, were given a series of reversal problems after having solved original discrimination. Although the lead-treated animals performed better than controls on the first reversal problems, their overall performance was significantly impaired in terms of errors made, thus essentially confirming the findings of Bushnell and Bowman (1979a).

Lilienthal *et al.* (1983, 1985) studied 'learning set formation (LSF)' according to Harlow (1949) in 17 rhesus monkeys. Six of them served as controls whereas eleven (5 low-Pb, 6 high-Pb) were given lead as lead acetate (190 and 320 mg/kg diet) starting *in utero* and extending until testing between about 30 and 50 months of age. Average PbB was below 10 µg/100 ml in controls and varied between 35 and 51 µg/100 ml in the low lead group and between 71 and 130 µg/100 ml in the high lead group. The animals were given a large number of discrimination problems varying in colour, form and size, which had to be solved successively. The number of trials necessary to solve each problem normally decreases with increasing number of trials; the animals, thus, 'learn how to learn'. Although no group differences occurred for simple discrimination learning across the first thirty problems, there were significant dose-related group differences for the formation of learning sets (Figure 15.2).

Even the inferiority of the low level animals as compared to control animals was significant. This study, again, confirms a NOEL below 35 μg/100 ml for primates.

The Reversibility-Issue

Only a few studies have addressed the question whether lead-induced behaviour-disorder persists after PbB has returned to pre-exposure levels upon cessation of lead exposure.

The study by Gross-Selbeck and Gross-Selbeck (1981) has already been described (p. 224). They demonstrated convincingly that elevated rates of bar pressing within an operant DRH schedule can still be detected in rats with only preweaning exposure after a decline of PbB from 20.5 μg/100 ml at weaning to 4.6 μg/100 ml at testing. This finding is suggestive of long-lasting behavioural effects of neonatal lead exposure.

Hastings *et al.* (1979) also exploited the neonatal exposure paradigm by giving lead (0.1 and 1 g/l) to lactating dams in drinking water. Lead exposure was discontinued at weaning when PbBs reached 29 and 65 μg/100 ml, respectively, with control levels around 11 μg/100 ml (see Table 15.1). At PND 120 the offspring were subjected to an operant simultaneous VDL task. A total of 96 per cent of controls, but only 63 per cent of the low-level group and 54 per cent of the high-lead group successfully learned to criterion; similar group differences occurred for days-to-criterion as the dependent variable. Although PbB was not measured at testing but was inferred from previous experience (Hastings *et al.*, 1977) to have declined to pre-exposure level, this study, again, confirms that behaviour deficit resulting from neonatal lead-exposure may extend into adult age.

Primate work bearing on the reversibility issue is also available, (Bushnell and Bowman, 1979b). Lead exposure of rhesus monkeys exposed from birth until twelve months of age (Bushnell and Bowman 1979a; see Table 15.1) was discontinued for 36 months. During this period PbBs, which had been 31.7 and 65.2 μg/100 ml for low- and high-lead groups, respectively, declined to a pre-exposure level around 5 μg/100 ml. At 49 months of age the animals were again placed on a discrimination reversal procedure with a set of new stimuli. Both lead groups required significantly more trials to reach criterion than controls. This deficit was

Figure 15.2: Learning Set-Formation in Rhesus Monkeys Pre- and Postnatally Exposed to Different Dietary Lead Levels; 0 (Controls), 190 (= 350 ppm), and 320 mg Pb/kg Diet (= 600 ppm). Percentage correct choices/trial in a two-choice task for the first six trials of all discrimination problems presented is given. Means and 95 per cent confidence limits are shown

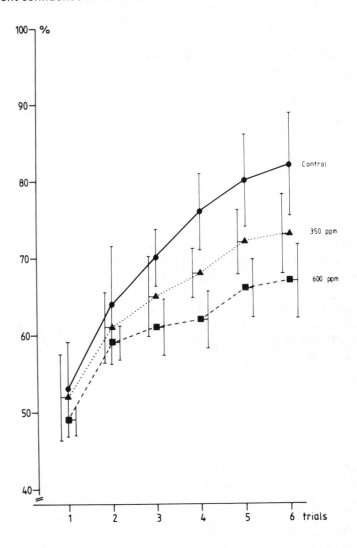

Source: Lilienthal *et al.* (1985)

apparent only for the first problem and nine reversals of it, whereas on subsequent problems no group differences occurred.

These studies, taken together, support the idea that lead exposure during early developmental stages may have long-lasting, perhaps irreversible, sequelae which can be detected by suitable behavioural tasks even when blood lead levels have returned to pre-exposure levels.

Lead and Animal Behaviour: Conclusions

Motor activity and learning are those behavioural dimensions which have received particular attention in studying the effects of inorganic lead on the nervous system of rats and monkeys.

As for motor activity there is sufficient evidence now to state with some certainty that hyperactivity or even increased activity is only secondary to lead exposure, and primarily related to lead-induced undernutrition during the early stages of brain development. This is not true for most of the more recent work on lead-related learning disorder. Most of the studies published since 1977 have avoided high levels of lead exposure so typical of the earlier work in this field and have, therefore, studied behavioural alterations in the absence of signs of overt toxicity, such as convulsions, weight loss or reduced litter size.

A wide variety of learning tasks, including negative and positive reinforcing contingencies, and ranging from shock-motivated avoidance learning to spatial and sensory discrimination learning, as well as to the multitude of operant techniques have been used in these studies. In terms of outcome this diversity of tasks has produced appreciable inter- and intra-task variability.

Spatial discrimination tasks have generally proved to be insensitive to the effects of lead, whereas visual discrimination learning (VDL) has given a rather consistent pattern of results, if task difficulty or task complexity was part of the study design. Examples of such strategies are the systematic variation of task difficulty in VDL studies on low-level effects of lead in rats (Winneke *et al.*, 1977, 1983), or the progression from simple VDL to discrimination reversal learning (Bushnell and Bowman, 1979a; Rice and Willes, 1979) or from simple VDL to higher-order learning in primates (Lilienthal *et al.*, 1983, 1985).

In some instances, such as in active avoidance learning

(Winneke *et al.*, 1982) or in operant DRH-tasks (Gross-Selbeck and Gross-Selbeck, 1981), as well as in fixed-interval schedules of reinforcement (Cory-Slechta and Thompson, 1979) it proved difficult to qualify observed lead effects as disorganised behaviour. It would seem, therefore, that the behaviour reflecting lead-induced alteration of normal neural functioning depends largely on the demand characteristics of the particular task. It may be disrupted as in difficult VDL tasks or adaptive as in tasks, in which speed of responding or disinhibition are reinforced.

The no-effect-level (NOEL) for behavioural effects in terms of blood lead concentrations still remains to be determined. For rats 17 µg/100 ml has so far been found as the lowest PbB associated with impaired learning performance (Winneke *et al.*, 1983), and several studies observed behavioural effects at PbBs between 20 and 30 µg/100 ml (Gross-Selbeck and Gross-Selbeck, 1981; Cory-Slechta and Thompson, 1979; Winneke *et al.*, 1977). In monkeys disruption of complex learning has been observed at PbBs ranging from 30 to 50 µg/100 ml.

It is still uncertain, however, how these values relate to blood lead levels in man. In terms of intake much higher lead doses are needed in the rat as compared to man to achieve comparable PbB levels. Schlipkoeter and Winneke (1980) have calculated from feeding studies that for a rat to reach PbBs between 15 and 18 µg/100 ml from dietary lead exposure, daily lead intake of about 60 mg/kg body weight is necessary assuming a daily food intake of 20 g for an adult rat. For man average daily lead intake of only about 7 µg/kg has been calculated (Lehnert *et al.*, 1969). This pronounced discrepancy is presumably related to differences in resorption as well as to a much shorter half-life of blood lead in rats as compared to man. These differences as well as those related to haem biochemistry, metabolism and other aspects of physiology limit the utility of the animal model for directly deriving dose-response functions applicable to the human condition.

It is important, however, that these animal studies have shown, that lead can be considered causative for neurobehavioural deficit, that, furthermore, such deficit is observed in the absence of overt signs of toxicity, i.e. in 'asymptomatic animals', and that some of the neurobehavioural deficit resembles cognitive deficit in man. Another important aspect of these animal studies is their contribution to the irreversibility problem. Although only a few studies have specifically addressed this issue, these have shown convincingly that the effect of neonatal preweaning lead exposure can still be detected in adult animals, whose blood lead levels have returned to pre-exposure levels after discontinuation of exposure.

The mechanism for this persistence of lead effects is not yet clarified, although the different kinetics of lead in brain tissue as compared to blood might serve as an explanation. Goldstein *et al.* (1974) have shown that lead enters the brain without threshold and that lead concentrations in the brain largely correspond to those in blood. After cessation of lead exposure PbB fell sharply whereas Pb levels in the brain did not change during the seven days post-exposure period. Hammond (1971) has shown, furthermore, that treatment with chelating agent, such as EDTA, causes lead excretion in the urine of young rats without a corresponding decrease in brain lead levels. There is additional evidence (Goldstein *et al.*, 1974) that lead is tightly bound to brain mitochondria and cannot be released by EDTA. These findings, taken together, may help us to understand why the neurobehavioural effects of early developmental lead exposure are long lasting or perhaps irreversible, as was shown in some of the animal studies covered in the present review.

References

Angell, N.F. and Weiss, B. (1982) Operant behavior of rats exposed to lead before or after weaning. *Toxicol. Appl. Pharmacol.*, *63*, 62-71.

Blackman, S.S., Jr (1937) The lesions of lead encephalitis in children. *Bull. Johns Hopkins Hosp.*, *61*, 1-43.

Bornschein, R., Pearson, D. and Reiter, L. (1980) Behavioral effects of moderate lead exposure in children and animal models: part 2, animal studies, *CRC Crit. Rev. Toxicol.*, *8*, 101-52.

Bushnell, P.J. and Bowman, R.E. (1979a) Reversal learning deficits in young monkeys exposed to lead, *Biochem. Behav.*, *10*, 733-42.

——, —— (1979b) Persistence of impaired reversal learning in young monkeys exposed to low levels of dietary lead, *J. Toxicol. Environ. Health*, *5*, 1015-23.

Castellano, C. and Oliverio, A. (1976) Early malnutrition and postnatal changes in brain and behavior in the mouse, *Brain Res.*, *101*, 317-20.

Cory-Slechta, D.A. and Thompson, T. (1979) Behavioral toxicity of chronic post-weaning lead exposure in the rat, *Toxicol. Appl. Pharmacol.*, *47*, 151-9.

——, Bissen, S.T., Young, A.M. and Thompson, T. (1981) Chronic postweaning lead exposure and response duration performance, *Toxicol. Appl. Pharmacol.*, *60*, 78-84.

Driscoll, J.W., Stegner, S.E. (1976) 'Behavioural effects of chronic lead ingestion on laboratory rats', *Pharmacol. Biochem. Behav.*, *4*, 411-17.

Environmental Protection Agency (EPA) (1977) *Air Quality Criteria for Lead* EPA-600/8-77-017. Government Printing Office, Washington, DC.

Goldstein, G.W., Asbury, A.K. and Diamond, I. (1974) Pathogenesis of lead encephalopathy: uptake of lead and reaction of brain capillaries, *Arch. Neurol.* (*Chicago*), *31*, 382-9.

Gross-Selbeck, E. and Gross-Selbeck, M. (1981) Changes in operant behavior of rats exposed to lead at the accepted no-effect level, *Clin. Toxicol.*, *18*, 1247-56.

Hammond, P.B. (1971) The effects of chelating agents on the tissue distribution and excretion of lead, *Toxicol. Appl. Pharmacol.*, *18*, 296-310.

Harlow, H.F. (1949) The formation of learning sets, *Psychol. Rev.*, *56*, 51-65.

Hastings, L., Cooper, G.P., Bornschein, R.L. and Michaelson, I.A. (1977) Behavioral effects of low level neonatal lead exposure, *Pharmacol. Biochem. Behav.*, *7*, 37-42.

—, —, — and — (1979) Behavioral deficits in adult rats following neonatal lead exposure, *Neurobehav. Toxicol.*, *1*, 227-31.

Krigman, M.A. and Hogan, E.L. (1974) Effect of lead intoxication on the post-natal growth of the nervous system, *Environ. Health Perspectives*, *7*, 187-99.

Lehnert, G., Stadelmann, G., Schalter, K.H., Szadkowski, D. (1969) 'Usuelle Bleibelastung durch Nahrungsmittel und Gehränke', *Arch. Hyg.*, *153*, 403-2.

Lilienthal, H., Winneke, G., Brockhaus, A., Molik, B. and Schlipkoeter, H.W. (1983) Learning set-formation in rhesus monkeys pre- and postnatally exposed to lead, in *Heavy Metals in the Environment* CEP-Consultants Edinburgh, pp. 901-3.

—, —, — and — (1985) Pre- and post-natal lead-exposure in monkeys: Effects on activity and learning set formation, *Neurobehav. Toxicol. Teratol.* (in press).

Milar, K.S., Krigman, M.R. and Grant, L.D. (1981) Effects of neonatal lead exposure on memory in rat, *Neurobehav. Toxicol. Teratol.*, *3*, 369-73.

Overmann, S.R. (1977) Behavioral effects of asymptomatic lead exposure during neonatal development in rats, *Toxicol. Appl. Pharmacol.*, *41*, 459-71.

Pentschew, A. (1958) Intoxikationen. in F. Heneke (ed.) *Handbuch der speziellen pathologischen Anatomie und Histologie*, vol. 13 Springer, Berlin, pp. 1910-14.

Pentschew, A. (1965) Morphology and morphogenesis of lead encephalopathy, *Acta Neuropathol.*, *5*, 133-60.

Pentschew, A. and Garro, F. (1966) Lead encephalomyelopathy of the suckling rat and its implications on the porphyrinopathic nervous diseases: with special reference to the permeability disorders of the nervous system's capillaries, *Acta Neuropathol.*, *6*, 266-78.

Perlstein, M.A. and Attala, R. (1966) Neurologic sequelae of plumbism in children, *Clin. Pediatr.*,(*Philadelphia*), *5*, 292-8.

Petit, I.L., Alfano, D.P. (1979) Differential experience following developmental lead exposure: Effects on brain and behavior, *Pharmacol. Biochem. Behav.*, *11*, 165-71.

Rice, D.C. and Willes, R.F. (1979) Neonatal low-level lead exposure in monkeys (*M. fascicularis*): Effect on two-choice non-spatial form discrimination, *J. Environ. Pathol. Toxicol.*, *2*, 1195-203.

Sauerhoff, M.W. and Michaelson, I.A. (1973) Hyperactivity and brain catecholamines in lead-exposed developing rats, *Science*, (*Washington*), *182*, 1022-4.

Schlipkoeter, H.W. and Winneke, G. (1980) Behavioral studies on the effects of ingested lead on the developing central nervous system of rats, in *Environmental Quality of Life: Lead Environmental Research Programme* Commission of the European Communities, Brussels, Luxembourg, pp. 127-34.

Silbergeld, E.K. and Goldberg, A.M. (1973) A lead-induced behavioral disorder, *Life Sci.*, *13*, 1275-83.

Silbergeld, E.K. and Goldberg, A.M. (1974) Hyperactivity: A lead-induced behavior disorder, *Environ. Health Perspect.*, *7*, 227-32.

Smith, H.D., Baehner, H.L., Carney, T. and Majors, W.J. (1963) The sequelae of Pica with and without lead poisoning. A comparison of the sequelae five or more years later, *Am. J. Dis. Child.*, *105*, 609-16.

Taylor, D.H., Noland, E.A., Brubaker, C.M., Crofton, K.M. and Bull, R.J. (1982) Low level lead (Pb) exposure produces learning deficits in young rat pups, *Neurobehav. Toxicol. Teratol.*, *4*, 311-14.

Winneke, G., Brockhaus, A., Baltissen, R. (1977) Neurobehavioral and systemic effects of longterm blood lead-elevation in rats. I. Discrimination learning and open field-behavior, *Arch. Toxicol.*, *37*, 247-63.

——, Kraemer, U., Brockhaus, A., Ewers, U., Kujanek, G., Lechner, H. and Janke, W. (1983) Neuropsychological studies in children with elevated tooth lead concentrations. Part II: Extended study, *Int. Arch. Occup. Environ. Health*, *51*, 231-52.

——, Lilienthal, H. and Werner, W. (1982) Task dependent neurobehavioral effects of lead in rats, *Arch. Toxicol. Suppl.*, *5*, 84-93.

——, —— and Zimmermann, U. (1983) Neurobehavioral effects of lead and cadmium, in A.W. Hayes, R.C. Schnell and T.S. Miya (eds.) *Developments in the Science and Practice of Toxicology*, Elsevier, Amsterdam, pp. 85-95.

16 LEAD, INTELLIGENCE, ATTAINMENT AND BEHAVIOUR

Richard Lansdown

Introduction

For the purposes of this chapter it will be helpful to consider children in three categories:

(1) Those who have suffered frank poisoning, leading to encephalopathy (i.e. inflamation of the brain).
(2) Those whose body lead burden is such that, although they shown no symptoms of encephalopathy, their functioning is impaired. These are children with a moderately elevated lead concentration.
(3) Those whose level of lead has no appreciable effect.

'Lead encephalopathy' was a term first offered in the landmark studies of Tanquerel des Planches in 1839 (Dana, 1848). Signs of encephalopathy, hyperirritability, ataxia, convulsions and coma, have been associated with blood lead levels from 90 to 800 µg/100 ml. Among the first to note the frequency of the occurrence of lead encephalopathy in children were Thomas and Blackfan (1914).

Children who survive encephalopathy may be left with permanent neurological sequelae; studies suggest that cerebral changes include gross oedema and widespread focal vascular lesions, associated with the accumulation of exudate, along with capillary neurosis and thrombosis (Blackman, 1937). An example of a study of post-encephalopathic lead poisoning is that of Perlstein and Attala (1966) who reported on 425 children aged 9 months to 8 years. Of the 59 with encephalopathy 89 per cent experienced some permanent neurological deficit: recurrent seizures and mental retardation were frequent.

It should be noted in this context that studies of children with very high levels of lead indicate the enormous variation in individuals. Some suffer irreversible brain damage or even death at levels of around 100 µg/100 ml, whereas others appear to show no effect at levels double this. The variation may be due to individual differences in susceptibility, changes in levels over time, increased tolerance for gradually accumulating burdens or interacting factors such as nutritional state.

Work involving encephalopathy attracts little controversy and results are generally quoted with confidence. However, fierce and often acrimonious debate surrounds studies concerned with moderately elevated levels, generally meaning those looking at the effects of lead when in the range up to 50 or 60 µg/100 ml. In essence the crucial questions are (a) does moderately elevated lead have an observable effect on behaviour and intelligence? and (b) is there a 'safe' level, below which no effect will be predicted? Because children are seen as particularly vulnerable to cerebral insult they have been the focus of much study.

For many years it was assumed that the then current levels of lead were below the safety threshold. Certainly children with pica were likely to ingest abnormal amounts of lead from old paint, or from sucking lead soldiers, but there was virtually no concern that the general population was at risk. One of the earliest warnings came from Patterson (1965) who argued that the average American had one hundred times the amount of lead in his body than would have been the case in a state of nature. Danielson (1970) questioned the hitherto accepted safety threshold of 80 µg/100 ml and in Great Britain Bryce-Smith (1971a) drew attention to recent evidence on general population lead levels, asserting that in some cases they exceeded concentrations at which metabolic processes can occur. Bryce-Smith drew particular attention to the dangers of increased mental retardation in children with moderately raised levels and, in a subsequent paper (1971b), to the possibility that some illness among the general population may be attributable to the present levels of lead.

The twenty years following Patterson's 1965 publication saw a steady increase in the number of studies, the quality of work and the level of passion as the arguments about safety, thresholds and the effects of current levels raged in the popular press as well as the scientific literature. The rest of this chapter will review the work available, from the 1940s to the present.

There have been three major literature reviews published recently and the work of their authors is acknowledged. In order of publication they were: Rutter (1980), Bornschein, Pearson and Reiter (1980) and Yule and Rutter (1985).

Summary of Major Published Studies on Lead, Intelligence and/or Behaviour

Reference	Population	n L: lead C: controls	Age	Blood or Tooth Lead	Main Results
De la Burdé and Choate (1972)	Inner city USA	L: 70 C: 72	4 4	40-100 not known	c sig. higher IQ
De la Burdé and Choate (1975)	Follow up of 1972	L: 70 C: 67	7 7	see above	c sig. higher IQ and sig. better on neurol. examination
Ernhart *et al.* (1981)	Inner city USA	L: 32 C: 31	8-13	32.4 ± 5 21.3 ± 4	c sig. higher IQ NS diff. on reading or behav. rating
Harvey *et al.* (1983)	Urban UK	189	2.5	15.5	NS diff. IQ or activity level.
Kotok (1972)	Inner city USA	L: 24 C: 25	x̄ : 2.8 x̄ : 2.7	58-137 20-55	NS diff. on developmental scale
Kotok *et al.* (1977)	Inner city USA	L: 31 C: 36	x̄ : 3.6	61-200 11-40	c sig. better on spatial tests; NS diff. on all other ability classes
Landrigan *et al.* (1975[a])	Smelter area USA	L: 78 C: 46	x̄ : 8.3 x̄ : 9.3	40-68 40	when 2 IQ tests combined c sig. higher, c sig. better on some neurological tests
Perino and Ernhart (1974)	Inner city USA	L: 30 C: 50	3-6	40-70 10-30	c sig. higher IQ
McBride *et al.* (1982)	Urban and surburban Australia	Moderate c.100 Low c.100	4.5 4.5	19-30 0.5-9	c sig. better on 2 out of 6 tests. NS diff. on other 4. NS diff. on activity scale
McNeil *et al.* (1975)	Smelter area USA	L: 23-161 C: 61-152	Mdn 9	40 40	NS diff. IQ, motor or vis. perceptual test. c sig. better on personality test
Needleman *et al.* (1979)	General pop. Urban USA	L: 58 C: 100	7 7	PbT: >24 ppm PbT: < 6ppm	c sig. better IQ and teachers' behaviour ratings
Ratcliffe (1977)	Smelter area UK	L: 24 C: 23	4-8 4-7	44.4 28.2	NS. differences develop. test or visual perception

Rummo et al. (1979)	Inner city USA	short Pb: 15 $\bar{x}$: 5.6 long Pb: 20 $\bar{x}$: 5.6 Post enc: 10 $\bar{x}$: 5.3 Control: 45 $\bar{x}$: 5.8		61 ± 7 68 ± 13 88 ± 40 23 ± 8	C < short Pb IQ Post enc < long Pb, < control. all Pb < 40 sig. higher IQ than all Pb > 40
Smith et al. (1983)	Urban UK	Hi: 155 Med: 103 Low: 145	6-7 6-7 6-7	PbT: $\bar{x}$ 11 µg/g PbT: $\bar{x}$: 6 µg/g PbT: $\bar{x}$: 3 µg/g	NS. diff. after adjusting for social factors on IQ, behaviour or attainment
Winneke et al. (1982)	Smelter area Duisburg FRG	L: 26 C: 26	8 8	PbT $\bar{x}$: 9.22ppm PbT $\bar{x}$: 2.4ppm	NS. diff. IQ, neurological test, behav. c sig. better on shape copying
Winneke et al. (1983)	Smelter area Stolberg FRG	89	9.4	PbT: 6.16ppm PbB: 14.3 µg	After adjusting for social factors NS. diff. IQ neurological test, behav. c sig. better on shape copying
Yule et al. (1981, 1983)	Urban UK	Gp 1:20 Gp 2:29 Gp 3:29 Gp 4:21	9 9 8 8	8.8 11.6 14.5 19.6	Sig. diff. IQ, reading, spelling and behav; low leads better than hi. NS. diff. maths
Yule et al. (1983)	Urban UK	80 82	9 9	7-12 13-24	NS. diff. on IQ, behav., attainment

Chelation study

David et al. (1983)	Groups	n[a]	$\bar{x}$ age	Blood leads		Hyperactivity within group change
				Baseline	Week 12	
Not known cause						
Penicillamine	26.31		7.4	28.5	19.8	sig. reduction
Methylphenidate	10-12		7.4	28.4	26.6	sig. reduction
Placebo	9-11		7.8	26.3	24.3	NS.
History of Lead Poisoning						
Penicillamine	13-14		8.6	35.0	25.7	sig. reduction

Note: [a] The numbers changed during the study. In the original report three tables are presented, each with different n values.

In the discussion in the rest of this chapter, the material has been divided into two sections, the first examining intelligence and attainment, and the second considering behaviour. To some extent this division is artificial, since both measured intelligence and overt behaviour are more or less functions of neurological states and many of the studies reviewed in the following pages deal with both. However, the distinction has been made partly because some of the problems of measurements differ and partly because the separation so produced will, it is hoped, help to clarify some of the issues.

Lead, Intelligence and Attainment

This section should be read in conjunction with Chapter 14 on methodological and statistical issues.

Having read this section it might be helpful for the reader to bear in mind some of the methodological points there mentioned. This is an area where complexity appears to grow, making the drawing of conclusions an impossible task. In essence, though, it can be argued that there is one outstanding methodological point which explains all findings: if confounding variables have consistently distorted the simple, apparent, direct relationship between lead and outcome variables, then a million studies all pointing in that same direction have as much scientific validity as sounding brass or tinkling cymbal.

Very High Lead Levels Without Encephalopathy

One of the most frequently quoted studies in the literature is that of Byers and Lord (1943). Twenty children who had been admitted to hospital for lead intoxication, without encephalopathy, were followed up. All were considered to have made a complete recovery but all but one were experiencing difficulties with school work showing evidence of emotional problems and deficits in perceptual-motor function. The authors concluded:

> The normal processes of intellectual growth and development are thought to be due to processes of maturation taking place in the cortex. It seems likely, therefore, that the lead in the circulation of an infant in some way interferes with the changes normally occurring in the cortex and in a high percentage of

cases prevents the normal growth and development of the cortex.

Further support for the Byers and Lord position came from Smith *et al.*'s (1963) study. In a five year follow up they found that the mean IQ of a group who had lead poisoning without encephalopathy was 87 compared to a mean of 98 for a group with pica but without elevated lead concentrations. A group with a history of encephalopathy had a mean IQ of 80.

Against these two studies can be placed that of Sachs *et al.* (1978, 1982) which examined 100 children, 74 per cent of whom had had blood leads in excess of 100 µg/100 ml. (The range of the whole group was from 68 to an astonishingly high 365 µg.) All children had been treated before the onset of encephalopathy. When compared with 28 siblings no significant differences were found on a battery of psychological tests.

The work reviewed above is not without weaknesses. Byers and Lord used no control group and took no note of social factors. Sachs *et al.* reported that the difference of 7 IQ points on the verbal scale of the Wechsler Intelligence test, in favour of the siblings, was statistically not significant but they used a non-parametric test; a more powerful parametric test might have yielded a different level of significance. Nevertheless, these studies were concerned still with children having had greatly elevated levels of lead. The rest of this chapter is concerned with children in the 'grey area'; those whose lead levels are more or less above average without generally reaching the boundary associated with encephalopathy, that is up to 70 to 80 µg/100 ml.

Moderately Raised Lead Levels

Because of the ethical constraints on taking blood from children not thought on *a priori* grounds to be at risk there have been severe limitations on the design of studies in this field. Researchers have been forced to a large extent to take what is available in terms of subjects and geographical locations, a point that critics seem sometimes to overlook.

Types of Study.   The classification of studies used here follows that of Rutter (1980). He grouped them as follows:

(1) Clinic-type studies of children with known high levels.
(2) Studies of deviant children.
(3) Chelation studies, that is the examination of children who have had high levels but who were 'deleaded' by chelation techniques.
(4) Smelter studies, that is work concerned with children living near a known lead emitting source, usually industrial.
(5) General population studies.

Clinic-type Studies of Children with Known High Lead Levels

De la Burdé and Choate (1972) selected a group of 70 lead-exposed children from a cohort of 3400 taking part in the collaborative study on cerebral palsy, mental retardation and other sensory disorders of infancy and childhood at the Medical College of Richmond, Virginia. Children were determined to be possible subjects only if their mothers reported that they engaged in pica. Experimental subjects were then selected if they lived in delapidated housing, had positive urinary coproporphyrin levels and blood lead levels greater than 40 µg/100 ml. The 70 children thus chosen had a mean blood lead level of 58 µg/100 ml, with a range of 40-100. (The final sample was 67 since three children were found to have signs of CNS anomalies.) A control group of 72 was matched for age, sex, maternal IQ, SES, the number of siblings below 6 years of age and housing density. The blood lead levels of the controls were not known (but see the account of de la Burdé and Choate 1975, below). Tests given at 4 years of age showed the assumed higher lead children to have a Stanford Binet IQ deficit of about 5 points and to include more mentally retarded (9 per cent vs none).

The statistical analysis was based on frequencies with no indication of certain cut-off points and tests of significance were applied only to tails of the distributions, thus inflating the chance of obtaining a significant finding.

The authors concluded: '... Admittedly the differences found may be due to environmental factors other than lead.'

However, a crucial characteristic allowing such a conclusion is the extent to which the selected group actually differed in lead exposure. Later work, De la Burdé and Shapiro (1975) showed that a small sample of the control group had elevated lead levels themselves (a mean of 53 µg/100 ml) and that a history of pica did not differentiate the two groups if the controls lived in rehabilitated older housing. Against these points are data from a follow up study, De la Burdé and Choate (1975) which showed very large differences in the tooth leads of those from whom teeth were available: 207 μg/g vs 122 μg/g, for 29 and 32 children respectively. This latter study reported IQ differences of about 3 points (WISC) at 7 years. It also noted that the control group mothers' mean non-verbal IQ score was four points higher than the experimental group.

Kotok (1972) compared 24 very high lead children (mean 81 μg/100 ml; range 58 to 137 μg/100 ml) to some with only high leads (mean 38 μg/100 ml; range 20-53 μg/100 ml) and found no difference in the results from the Denver Developmental Screening Test. The high general level of leads, the lack of information on the lead exposure history of both groups and the crudity of the test used argue for a cautious interpretation of these data.

In a further, similar but somewhat more sophisticated study, Kotok *et al.* (1977) compared a study group of 31 children aged 3.5 years, mean blood lead level 76.9 μg/100 ml with 36 children matched for age and pica with a mean blood lead of 28.3 μg/100 ml. A battery of subtests taken from various scales was used and no significant differences were found between the two groups. On the one hand this may not be surprising given the high levels of the control group, 15 of whom were between 30 and 40 μg/100 ml. On the other hand it should be noted that the general trend was for the very high lead children to register lower scores, although the differences did not reach the 5 per cent level of significance. It remains difficult to generalise from either of these Kotok studies given the atypical nature of almost all the children concerned.

A further study of children with high levels was conducted (Rummo, 1974; Rummo *et al.*, 1979) in which 44 children attending a hospital clinic who had a minimum level of 40 μg/100 ml on at least two occasions were compared with 45 controls matched for neighbourhood, age, sex and race. The groups did not differ in terms of SES or pica although there were some differences, e.g. maternal IQ. Children were given the McCarthy Scales of Intelligence, the results being:

(1) Short-term exposure (n : 15, mean blood lead 61 μg/100 ml) mean Cognitive Index score 94.1 (The Cognitive Index is equivalent to an IQ.)

(2) Long-term exposure (n : 20, mean blood lead 68 μg/100 ml,

with high levels maintained for at least six months) mean Cognitive Index score 87.8.

(3) An encephalopathy group (n : 10, mean blood lead 88 μg/ 100 ml) mean Cognitive Index score 75.7.

(4) Controls (n : 45, mean blood lead 23 μg/100 ml) mean Cognitive Index score 93.3.

When the children were combined and divided according to blood lead level there was a clear distinction between the groups, the lowest leads ($<$ 40 μg) having a mean score of 92.7 compared to the highest (80+ μg) where the mean was 50.0. It is, incidentally, curious to note, as Rutter (1980) did, that the figures given in Rummo's original thesis differ slightly from those presented in the subsequent paper. The latter are given above.

These results undoubtedly point to the adverse effects of high lead levels and suggest a dose effect at those levels below the encephalopathy group. Further support for a subencephalopathy effect is found in the results which showed lead to be associated with slower reaction times and finger tapping and poor leg coordination. Rummo herself was perhaps excessively cautious, in view of the trends of these results, in saying that chronic low level lead exposure does not have effects similar to those of a higher exposure. In many ways this was a well-designed piece of work; it is unfortunate that maternal education was not used as a covariate and that no account was given of the history of the children's exposure to lead.

Albert *et al.* (1974) conducted a follow up study of New York children suspected of excessive lead exposure. A subsample, all above 7 years of age, was assessed on a battery of tests and were grouped according to their lead levels. Among the results it was found that three children in an encephalopathy group had a mean IQ of 77.0; 25 with blood leads above 60 μg/100 ml had a mean IQ of 92.4, whereas 39 controls, with lead levels below 60 μg had a mean IQ of 98.9. Despite the internal consistency of these results little weight can be attatched to them since only 40 per cent of the children were traced and there was inadequate matching on socioeconomic variables.

Baloh *et al.* (1975) looked at 27 asymptomatic children, mean age 5.5 years, who had at least two blood lead levels above 50 μg/ 100 ml, comparing them with a similar number of controls matched for age, sex, race and SES. The groups did not differ significantly on measures of IQ or tests of fine motor ability. There are, however, some puzzling aspects of this study: six of the 27 controls had lead levels between 30 and 40 µg/100 ml at the time of testing and the mean level of the study children at testing had fallen to 44 µg/100 ml. It is uncertain where the high lead children obtained their lead from and there is the possibility that the controls had higher levels when young.

A not dissimilar design was used by Needleman (1977) when he compared 41 six to eight year-old boys in Boston who had one or more level of 50 µg/100 ml or more with 35 comparable boys who had never had levels above 30 µg/100 ml. Few of the test results reached statistical significance and although there was some support for the general notion of a falling off in performance at levels above 50 µg conclusions must be tentative in view of the large number of children not followed up and the long gap between blood lead testing and the administration of the psychological battery.

Conclusions.   The studies in this section generally point in the same direction although none is without flaws and all are open to alternative interpretations. The direction is that moderately elevated lead levels, that is in the 60+ µg/100 ml are likely to be associated with a small reduction in IQ, perhaps of 3-4 points. Conclusions on children with concentrations between 40 and 60 are less clear and little can be said with certainty on children in the ranges up to 15 µg/100 ml.

Studies of Mentally Retarded Children

The general conceptual approach of these studies is simple and at first appealing. Children with known retardation are compared with others and if the former have higher lead levels it may be concluded that lead is a causal factor. Unfortunately, as has been discussed in Chapter 14, the picture is not as simple as that: so often lead may be no more than a marker for another factor.

One of the earliest studies in this area was that of Moncrieff *et al.* (1964). Nearly half the group of 122 retarded children had blood lead levels above 36 µg/100 ml. Immediately one comes up against the methodological problem noted above: it is known that mentally retarded children have a high incidence of pica and it is possible that their higher levels of lead, obtained perhaps from chewing painted surfaces, was a result rather than a cause of their retardation.

The work of Gibson *et al.* (1967) confirms the possible validity of this interpretation of Moncrieff's findings. Three groups of children, 20 in each group were compared. The first were retarded with a known aetiology: none had blood lead levels above 40 μg/ 100 ml. The second were retarded but with no known aetiology: six had levels above 40 μg/100 ml. The third were children with orthopaedic or cardiac disorders: three had levels above 40 μg/ 100 ml. The inference from these findings could be that lead was a causal factor in the retardation of the second group but it was noted that all the children with high lead levels showed pica and all but one lived in old houses. The children with retardation of known aetiology were less mobile than the others and so possibly had restricted access to lead.

It is known that a combination of soft water and lead pipes is likely to increase lead intake (see Chapter 9) and the hypothesis that this has given rise to mental retardation was tested by Beattie *et al.* (1975) in Glasgow. Higher amounts of lead were found in the water in the homes of mentally retarded children than in those of controls from the same area. Since the lead in those cases was found in water, pica cannot be invoked to explain the differences. However, although this study is provocative, matching was not perfect and it is possible that there was some bias in the sampling. Set against the Glasgow work is that of Elwood *et al.* (1976) which was carried out in Wales: Beattie's findings were not replicated. It must not be assumed, though, that the Welsh finding necessarily contradicts that of Beattie *et al.* since the lead levels in Wales were well below those in Glasgow.

In an attempt to avoid pica or any other behavioural variables Moore *et al.* (1977) looked at phenylketonuria (PKU) cards to examine the blood lead levels of new-born children. The mean levels of those found subsequently to be retarded were higher than those of the controls. Unfortunately a high proportion of the PKU cards could not be traced and this study remains interesting but inconclusive.

Pihl and Parkes (1977) looked at the hair metal content of 31 learning-disabled children compared to 22 controls from the same school, and found large differences between the groups for many metals including lead. This result is difficult to interpret partly because the measurement of lead in hair is a dubious activity and partly because the authors' definition of learning disabled precluded clear identification of the children's cognitive deficits.

The most often quoted work in this area is that of David and his colleagues, much of which has been concerned with hyperactive children and which will be reviewed later in this chapter. David *et al.* (1976) used a design similar to that of Gibson *et al.* (1967). The mean blood levels for mentally retarded children of unknown aetiology (25.5 µg/100 ml) was markedly higher than that of the children with aetiology probably known (18.7 µg) or a control group (18.8 µg). However, little is reported on the social background of the children and no data are available on pica, rendering the work much less valuable than it might have been.

Conclusions. While several of the studies quoted above give results in the same general direction they should not *ipso facto* be seen as supporting the causal relationship between lead and mental retardation. If, as is possible, they share certain methodological weaknesses they may simply be reflecting consistent design and interpretation errors.

Chelation Studies

Observations from experiments in which one variable can be manipulated are considerably more powerful than those in which only associations can be examined. In human studies ethical constraints forbid the manipulation of most variables but chelation, a technique used to reduce the amount of lead in the body, is an exception in that it is ethically possible and may even be desirable in some cases. If some high lead children could be shown to have increased in IQ scores when the only before and after difference was one of lead reduction much of the doubt about causality would be removed.

However, work on animals (see Chapter 15) suggests that a reduction of lead in the body does not necessarily mean that there will be a comparable reduction in the brain. The problem of irreversibility may, indeed, be such that chelation studies will not produce as conclusive an answer as might at first have seemed likely.

Rutter (1980) has pointed out that such studies should meet the following criteria.

(1) Contrasting interventions should be used to test whether the

change observed is related only to a lead effect or whether it derives from a general therapeutic contact.

(2) The use of either a control group or adequate baseline periods to ensure that recorded gains in IQ are not due to normal fluctuation or changes related to experience.

Unfortunately none of the published studies on chelation and IQ meets these criteria. Pueschel *et al.* (1972) reported a rise in IQ of eight points among 35 out of 58 children treated but no control group was used.

The work of Sachs *et al.* (1978, 1982) has already been mentioned above, when the results and weaknesses of their studies were discussed.

Kirkconnell and Hicks (1980) selected 22 children from a pool of those chelated and compared their scores on the Denver Developmental Screening Test with 22 controls matched for age and socioeconomic background. The ratio scores, i.e. the scores corrected for age, remained constant for the controls, as would be predicted, over a period of 18 months. The treated-group's ratio scores fell during the 25 months following chelation. The authors argue for a residual lead effect; it is certainly unlikely that lead had increased IQ but haphazard sampling and the use of a crude developmental measure reduce confidence in either interpretation.

Conclusion.   The use of chelation may remain a powerful means of examining lead and intellectual development but it has not yet been fully exploited. (See also the relevant part in the section on behaviour later in this chapter.)

Smelter Studies

One of the earliest studies to examine the association between elevated lead levels and intelligence among children living around a known source of lead was that of Lansdown *et al.* (1974). Data were obtained on 232 children living in London and no relationship was found between a single blood lead level taken some time before and IQ, or between the distance of the children's homes from the factory and IQ. The absence of data on the children's social background and the suggestion that the low lead group came from more deprived families (Lansdown, 1977) weaken conclusions to be drawn from these data.

A series of studies was undertaken by several workers on

children living in the vicinity of a lead-emitting smelter in El Paso. Landrigan *et al.* (1975a, b) divided children into two groups using blood lead samples collected in 1972: the high lead group had levels from 40-80 μg/100 ml, the others were below 40 μg. All children were asymptomatic and the groups were matched on half a dozen key variables including length of residence and proximity to the smelter. By 1973 blood lead levels still showed a difference between the two groups although almost half the high leads had fallen to below 40. There was no difference between the two on verbal IQ although the performance IQ was lower among the higher lead children (95 vs 103).

Several factors within the study lead to a critical appraisal of the results. The children whose lead levels fell did no better than those whose levels remained high; reliance on a single measure to differentiate the groups may have masked a greater similarity between the two than was apparent; there was an unexplained verbal-performance discrepancy in the controls which accounted for the IQ differences.

McNeil *et al.* (1975) worked in the same area but used different samples and a different research design. The experimental group was defined in terms of proximity to the smelter and were matched on age, sex, ethnic background and family income with controls. Mean blood lead differences were significant (50 μg/100 ml vs 20 μg). No differences were found on measures of IQ or teachers' report; the performance scores were 95 vs 93. In many ways this is a convincing study: the authors' caution in their interpretation of the negative results adumbrated much that has been suggested later, i.e. the high level of nourishment of the El Paso children might have been a protective factor offsetting potential lead effects. However, the finding that there was no apparent difference in scores of children whose lead levels were as disparate as 60 μg or more compared to those with a mean level of 26 is puzzling in that it is so much against the trend in the literature. This point, coupled with a different result from that reported by Landrigan, poses a question mark over the El Paso results in general.

Hebel *et al.* (1976) reported on the attainment scores of 11-year-old children in Birmingham according to the distance of their homes from a factory making batteries. No differences were found as a function of proximity but since no data on lead levels were available the results are inconclusive.

Ratcliffe (1977) found consistent differences *in favour* of a

5-year-old 'moderate' lead group living near a lead battery factory in Manchester, compared to a high lead group (means of 28 μg and 44 μg/100 ml) on tests of intelligence, behaviour and visual perception. However, the differences were not statistically significant and the estimates of blood lead levels were made 3 years before the psychological testing.

As part of the Idaho study (Wegner, 1976), Gregory *et al.* (1976) tested children between 5 and 10 years of age living around a smelter. There were consistent but not always significant differences in WISC scores and a correlation of −0.182 between IQ and lead after partialling out the effect of socioeconomic status. There are several aspects to this study which qualify its acceptance. Tester effects were found (i.e. one tester out of a total of six was discrepant) which may have minimised the observed differences; there was a high loss of potential subjects; there were no data on parental IQ; information on lead exposure history is sketchy.

Conclusion. The overall results of smelter studies have been disappointing. Results have conflicted, numbers are often small and background information is often missing. Taken together their main contribution is to the realisation of the complexity of the subject they are addressing.

General Population Studies

Tooth Lead Measures. Since the late 1970s attention has turned to data obtained from large samples drawn at random from the general population. A consideration of the methodological advantages and pitfalls of this approach is given in Chapter 14. One of the pioneers in this field is Needleman, who with co-workers in Massachusetts produced one of the most influential studies in the literature (Needleman *et al.*, 1979).

Shed deciduous teeth were collected by teachers in first and second grades (6 and 7 year olds) in the schools of two towns. Of the population of 3329 eligible children 70 per cent gave teeth in return for a badge. Children were excluded if they came from homes where English was not the first language, if they were not born at term, had a health history indicating noteworthy head injury or had unco-operative parents. This accounted for about half the eligible children. A mean tooth lead concentration of 14.03 ppm was found and two groups created from the highest 10 per cent ($>$ 24 ppm, n $=$ 58) and lowest 10 per cent ($<$ 6 ppm, n $=$ 100), on the basis of two concordant dentine samples.

The children were then given a four hour battery of tests during which time the mother completed a questionnaire to yield background information and a picture vocabulary test to give an estimate of maternal IQ. Teachers submitted a behaviour rating, which is discussed along with other studies on behaviour later in this chapter.

Some validation of the tooth lead levels was found from an examination of the blood lead levels taken from a proportion of the children four to five years earlier. Of the high lead children 23 had a mean blood level of 35.5 µg/100 ml (range 18 to 54) compared to the low tooth lead group's mean of 23.8 (range 12 to 37). Five variables differentiating the two groups were noted as covariates and after analysis of covariance the corrected mean IQs were 106.6 for the low lead group compared to 102.1 for the high group, a statistically significant difference. There was a similar trend throughout the extensive battery of tests with a striking effect on reaction times. In a subsequent report (Needleman *et al.*, 1982) the point was made that the average IQ deficit in this study did not reflect only impairment in children with already low IQs; rather the entire distribution of IQ in the high lead group was shifted downwards.

Needleman's study has been the centre of a fierce controversy. The design was weak in that a middle group was omitted, so that it was not possible to examine a dose effect properly. The behaviour rating results are impressive at first glance but they are not corrected for social factors or for IQ. The large number of excluded families might have introduced a certain bias into the final sample and no attempt appears to have been made to control for variations in lead levels of teeth by type or position in the mouth, a factor which Smith *et al.* (1983) found of great importance.

The criticisms noted above were apparent on the publication of the paper. Subsequently the American Environmental Protection Agency commissioned an examination of the work (Marshall, 1983). This examination resulted in suggestions that the Needleman computer program contained errors, and there were questions on the controls for confounding variables and the method for selecting the sample.

Following these suggestions Needleman's data were reworked

and presented at an EPA meeting held in North Carolina in April 1984 with the general conclusion that the changes in analyses made no difference to the overall results offered in the original paper.

A series of studies similar to those of Needleman have been carried out in Germany by Winneke and colleagues. The first, a pilot, was conducted in Duisburg, an industrial city with known heavy air pollution, in 1976 (Winneke *et al.*, 1982). Deciduous teeth were collected in a press-supported campaign from 1238 children but only 458 were included in the sample, the criteria being that they had given at least two incisor teeth and were representative of the general population. Tooth lead levels ranged from 1.4 to 12.7 ppm with a geometric mean of 4.6 ppm. Those children with concentrations below 3 ppm were called the low group, those above 7 ppm the high group. Children whose parents agreed to take part were then matched for age, sex and social class and 26 matched pairs were then tested on a battery including the German version of the WISC. There were consistent differences between the pairs in favour of the low lead children, for example the full scale IQs were 130 and 123. (The very high WISC score probably reflects an out of date standardisation.) None of the differences reached statistical significance and the results were seen as no more than suggestive.

Winneke's next, more extensive study set out to include more children and to take note of more social variables. It was carried out in Stolberg, (Winneke et al., 1983) a small industrial city; 338 children (less than 10 per cent of the possible 3669 whose parents were asked to co-operate) gave teeth. After the discarding of teeth unsuitable for analysis, 317 children remained in the study. Further exclusions, e.g. of non-German children, reduced the numbers once more and the final tested groups were Low ($<$ 4.2 ppm), Middle (5.8-7.2 ppm) and High ($>$ 9.8 ppm). The geometric mean was 6.2 ppm. A total of 115 children were tested, with a mean age of 9.4 years. The mean blood lead from a subsample of 83 children was 14.3 µg/100 ml and the correlation between teeth and blood measures was +0.47 ($P < 0.01$).

A battery of tests was given and mothers took part in a semi-standardised interview to obtain background information.

Before corrections for confounding variables the difference between the verbal IQ of the high and the low groups was 7.6 points in favour of the latter; after correction it fell to 4.6 points. Neither difference was statistically significant. The problem was similar for the full scale IQ but less marked for the performance scores. The middle group fell between the two extremes but tended to be nearer the 'low' children.

Further analyses (Winneke and Kramer, 1983) suggested that certain perceptuo-motor measures and reaction times showed an association between raised lead levels and impaired functioning only for the subgroup of socially disadvantaged children. This finding did not apply to IQ results.

The Stolberg study has many strong points. The lead levels were more in line with ordinary current exposure than those of Needleman and the inclusion of a middle group was a further advantage. However, the sample size was small for a study of this nature, and the analyses were based on only a small proportion of the overall population (only 10 per cent of children gave teeth and one quarter of the eligible families were unwilling to participate in the study).

The most recently published epidemiological study using tooth lead as an index of exposure had the advantage of being able to overcome many of the methodological problems encountered by Needleman and Winneke. Smith *et al.* (1983) invited children from three London boroughs to donate teeth, using a badge as a reward, and three-fifths of the total population of 6875 gave at least one tooth. The children were in their last year of infant education (aged 6-0 to 6-11 years at the start of the school year) and those who were not native born of non-immigrant families or who had any major physical or emotional disability were excluded. This was the first study carefully to denominate the whole population, thus allowing the authors to describe the characteristics of tooth givers vs non-tooth givers. As might be expected, the former tended to be of a slightly higher social class, included more girls, scored higher on tests of attainment and were better behaved. Although all these differences were small they were statistically significant. Three groups were selected from those eligible, to form high (n: 155), medium (n: 103) and low (n: 145) lead groups with clearly differentiated differences in tooth lead content of $\geqslant 8$ ppm, 5-5.5 ppm and $\leqslant 2.5$ ppm respectively. A total of 97 per cent of parents of eligible children agreed to co-operate.

An extensive family interview was carried out, including observations on the children's homes and a measure of maternal IQ. Children's lead levels were significantly associated with family cleanliness, the presence of peeling paint, mothers' smoking, pica, the nature of habitual play space, proximity to a waste ground, demolition and building sites and diet. There was no association with proximity of home or school to a main road.

A battery of tests was given, with no significant differences between the groups being found on any of these cognitive measures: Seashore rhythm test, visual and auditory memory, shape copying and reaction time. However, the IQ results were significantly different with mean scores as follows: high lead group: 103.7, medium: 104.9 and low: 108.7.

Scores on reading and maths were obtained on all children who gave teeth and both showed a trend for the higher lead children to have lower scores.

The family interviews yielded sufficient data to allow for sophisticated controlling of factors which might have produced an artefactual association between lead levels and outcome variables. As a result of this the differences in scores noted above were all reduced and while the trend remained in the same direction statistical significance was no longer reached on any outcome measure.

This is one of the best designed, most extensive studies so far published and the basic findings can be accepted as valid. However, some minor points warn against a wholesale acceptance of the generalisability of the findings: the sample was slightly biased towards the socially advantaged, the non-significant differences remaining after controlling for social variables might, in fact, be lead related. Taking up this latter point: the choice of control by concomitant variables that correlated only with outcome variables rather than the more conventional choice of variables correlating with both the independent variable and the outcome variable is not uncontroversial and has led some commentators, e.g. Yule and Rutter (1985), to conclude that there might have been a degree of overcorrection. If this latter view is accepted then the non-significant result found by Smith *et al.* could still reflect a lead effect. This was not the conclusion of the authors who summarised their discussion in an ultra cautious fashion: '. . . in environments similar to the one in which this research was carried out . . . it is uncertain whether measurable improvements in children's intelligence, educational attainment, behaviour etc. would result from a reduction in the body-lead burden of children'.

Blood Lead Studies.   Perino and Ernhart (1974) compared 30 asymptomatic New York children whose blood lead levels were in the range 40-70 µg/100 ml with 50 controls in the 10-30 µg range, matched for age, sex, socioeconomic status, birth weight and maternal IQ. Lead measures were taken two weeks before intelligence testing and the two showed a statistically significant association even with the control factors taken into account. The difference in scores on the McCarthy scale was higher than that usually reported: 90.14 vs 79.83. The correlation between parental and child IQ for the controls was the expected 0.52, while that for the exposed group was only 0.10.

Although this work has much to commend it, there are flaws. There was, for example, a significant negative correlation between lead level and parental educational level, i.e. the better-educated parents had children with less lead. It is possible that there was, then, a set of confounding variables affecting both lead exposure and performance on the intelligence test; without an adequate history of exposure it is not possible to be certain.

A recent follow up study Ernhart *et al.* (1981) re-examined 63 of the original sample and found the mean blood lead levels correlated positively (0.46) with those obtained earlier although the mean had dropped from 32.5 to 26.9. The concurrent blood lead measures continued to show a significant association with IQ although controlling for factors such as parental IQ reduced the association considerably. The authors concluded that these follow up findings were only a few of those also reported on, and that they could have arisen by chance. However, Ernhart *et al.*'s conclusions have not always been accepted; Yule and Rutter (1985) see these two New York studies as essentially supporting the notion that there is a small but significant association between lead and measured IQ in the ranges quoted. The Ernhart work is currently being reanalysed following the EPA enquiry noted above.

Support for the Yule and Rutter interpretation of Ernhart's work comes from a replication of the 1974 study by Yamin (1976). A total of 80 low social class black children with a mean blood lead level of 33 µg/100 ml (range 15-56) were assessed and lead was seen to contribute 2-3 per cent of the total variance of measures related to intelligence, after correction for social factors.

Four blood lead studies have recently been carried out in Britain. In the first (Yule *et al.*, 1981) children living near a battery works in London with blood lead levels ranging from 7 to 32 µg/ 100 ml, the mean being 13.5 µg, were given tests of intelligence and attainment. It is interesting to note the relatively low levels of lead even in this supposed 'at risk' group. After extensive analyses lead and IQ were correlated even after age, sex and social class were partialled out. There was a mean group difference of about 7 IQ points between the highest and the lowest lead quartiles, with a suggestion that a level of 12 µg/100 ml marked some form of threshold effect. A possibly very important point is that the 'lead effect' was observable only in children whose fathers had manual occupations (Yule *et al.*, 1983). This study was described by the authors as a pilot. It was mounted hurriedly with no time being available for extensive data collections on family variables.

Their second study (Yule *et al.*, 1983) was based on a group of London children whose blood lead levels had been assessed in 1980 at the request of their parents: the children's schools were in the vicinity of a busy road. Psychological testing and parent interviews (with a schedule based on that devised by Smith *et al.*) was carried out 20 months after the blood tests. Brief IQ measures were taken from both parents. There was an 88 per cent response rate.

The sample differed from the first in several respects. Three-fifths of the fathers were in non-manual occupations, compared to one-fifth; the mean blood lead level was slightly lower, 12.8 µg/ 100 ml compared to 13.5 µg/100 ml and there was no association between social class and lead level, although the non-significant trend was in the usual direction. As might be expected the children's attainment and IQ were above average and the rate of behaviour disturbance was low.

More striking was the difference in results in terms of the associations between lead, intelligence and attainment: in essence there was none. (For a discussion on behaviour see later in this chapter). There was a weak, non-significant association between lead and outcome measures in the working class group but none whatsoever in the majority of the children.

The reasons for the difference in outcome of these two studies is far from clear. The sample size was much the same, the test batteries identical; the second study yielded negative results before and after correction for social variables. The most likely explanation is that the two groups differed in social composition.

The third study in this series was carried out in Leeds, a city where there was excellent environmental data on lead and its sources. Over 300 children were given a battery similar to that used in the two London studies and the results have indicated no lead/IQ or attainment associations.

Almost all work in this field has been carried out with children of school age. An exception is that of Harvey *et al.* (1983), in which 189 children aged 30 months, born to European, English-speaking parents living in Birmingham, with a birth weight in excess of 2500 g formed the sample. A single blood lead measure gave a mean of 15.6 µg/100 ml with a standard deviation of 4.2. Parents were interviewed and mothers' IQ assessed with the Ravens Matrices and Mill Hill Vocabulary Test. Before correction for social variables the correlation between blood lead and childrens IQ was 0.17, after correction this correlation virtually disappeared. A possibly very important finding was the difference, before correction, in the correlations between lead and IQ as a function of social class: for the manual group it was 0.32, for the non-manual 0.06.

The social enquiry produced some unexpected results. Peeling paint, ordinal position within the family and mother's IQ were the three most powerful predictors of IQ but not of lead levels. There remains a lurking suspicion that somehow these variables are related to lead exposure although the thorough statistical analysis argues against such a conclusion. A further query remains over the sample: 46 per cent were not available and of those who were only 44 per cent could be tested.

Another recent study paying attention to social variables and young children is that of Milar *et al.* (1981) who assessed 52 asymptomatic children aged 10 to 73 months referred to a lead screening programme in North Carolina. Families of children with lead levels above 30 µg/100 ml were compared with those below this cut off figure. Caldwell and Bradley's (1978) Home Observation for Measurement of the Environment (HOME) inventory, plus maternal IQ were used. There were differences in results according to the age of the child.

In the younger (below 30 months) group the HOME scores were worse and the maternal IQ scores lower in the high lead group. The differences were less marked, falling short of statistical significance, in the older group.

The only other study so far published in this area was that of McBride *et al.* (1982). About 200 children aged 4 to 5 living in

Sydney were studied. Of the population approached 37 per cent failed to reply and 3 per cent refused to participate. Blood lead levels averaged 14 µg/100 ml with a range from 0.5 to 30 and over one-third of the fathers had professional or managerial occupations. There was no association between lead and performance in a picture vocabulary test and various measures of motor function.

Other Investigation. Thatcher *et al.* (1982) recruited 149 rural American school children through newspaper advertisements and had hair analysed. The children were then divided into quartiles according to their hair analysis and regression analyses showed that hair lead was significantly associated with Wechsler IQs after controlling for age, sex, race and socioeconomic status. The findings are consistent with many other studies but the use of hair as a marker for lead remains controversial.

Verbal or Performance Effects. As was noted in Chapter 14, the Wechsler Scales yield results that enable one to make inferences about different aspects of children's ability, most commonly there is an expression of verbal scores and performance, or non-verbal scores. The McCarthy scales yield similar patterns. One of the striking results of several studies using such tests is that verbal rather than performance scores are depressed. Needleman *et al.* (1979), Perino and Ernhart (1974), Ernhart *et al.* (1981), Yule *et al.* (1981) and Winneke *et al.* (1983) all reported results in this direction.

On the other hand this has not been a consistent finding, indeed one of the puzzling sets of findings from various studies has been the lack of consistency in type of deficit. This was most apparent in the Needleman *et al.* (1979) study and its subsequent partial replications by Yule *et al.* (1981, 1983) and Smith *et al.* (1983). The lead effect came and went, now appearing on one test, now on another, here on almost all, there on almost none. One is forced to conclude that if there is an effect at low to moderate levels there must be powerful interactions with factors related to individual differences between children.

General Conclusions. Much doubt remains but recent studies, particularly those carried out in Great Britain, have gone some way towards clarifying certain issues.

The first point to bear in mind is that the effect of lead on intelligence if it exists at all within the range of lead burdens experienced by the general population of children, is small. Most studies have pointed to a difference of up to about 5 or 6 IQ points, with data suggesting that lead accounts for no more than 2 or 3 per cent of the variance in cognitive performance. This is much less than is accounted for by genetic and many other environmental factors. However, small is a relative term and as several commentators have pointed out, a *population* shift of 5 IQ points up or down is not negligible.

The second is that the recent epidemiological work in Britain, Germany and the USA has all pointed in the same direction. The body of large-scale surveys suggests at least a possibility that lead is causally related to deficits in cognitive functioning.

The third point is hardly a conclusion since it has only recently been raised. Much of the early investigation of this whole area was conducted on mainly socially disadvantaged children. The more recent studies in Britain and Germany have suggested that there may be virtually no causal relationship among children from more advantaged homes. If this finding is found to have a scientific basis it may go a long way towards explaining some of the apparent contradictions in earlier work.

Little has been said about a possible threshold effect or 'safe' level of lead, possibly because the notion of a clear cut-off point is questionable: for some commentators even a concentration of 7 µg/100 ml might be seen as dangerous. This point is taken up further in Chapter 17.

Lead and Behaviour

Many chemical substances are known to affect behaviour. Alcohol, tranquillisers and antidepressants are those which possibly spring to mind most readily.

The nature of behavioural abnormalities associated with moderately raised lead levels is widespread. Bryce-Smith (1972) was one of the earliest to argue that subtle disturbances of behaviour might be manifest long before any classical symptoms of poisoning are apparent.

In studies on adults the following effects have been reported: excitement, restlessness, agitation, insomnia, nightmares, impairment of memory, loss of concentration, low sexual potency, constipation, headaches and depression (Bryce-Smith, 1972). This (suspiciously over-inclusive) list is seen by the author to reflect disturbances primarily in the autonomic nervous system. Children, he argues, are more sensitive to lead than adults and the central nervous system is more seriously involved. The behavioural abnormality most often associated with moderately raised levels of lead in children is that cluster related to attention: easy distractibility, poor concentration, overactivity, dreaminess, impulsiveness. This last point has been seized on, e.g. by Bryce-Smith and Waldron (1974), to provide a partial explanation for many delinquent acts including football hooliganism. 'Offenders of this type would be better treated with penicillamine than prison.' (Penicillamine is a chelating, or 'de-leading' agent.) It must, however, be pointed out that a word of caution is added: 'just as we have emphasised that lead is by no means the only important factor in behaviour disturbance, so do we also emphasise that hyperactivity is not the only factor in criminality'.

The rest of this chapter consists of a review of those studies addressing themselves to behavioural factors alleged to be associated with lead levels not sufficiently high to cause encephalopathy. Those which have already been described in the first part of this chapter will be mentioned first and readers are asked to refer to the above section for an account of the sample and methodological characteristics of each study. Page references are given to facilitate this cross reference.

Studies Already Outlined Earlier in this Chapter

Clinic-type Studies. The first (Byers and Lord (1943) p. 239) referred to teachers' complaints of the children's 'inattention and restlessness' but no formal assessment of behaviour was undertaken.

De la Burdé and Choate (1972) (p. 241) confirmed this conclusion with rather more convincing measures. Children were rated on ten five-point scales and assigned to various categories. Extreme negativity, distractability and a constant need for attention were found as a triad to be more common among the lead-exposed children than the controls and the former were shown to have a greater chance of having at least one behavioural deficit.

However, five subsequent studies failed to confirm the picture, although not all dismissed the effects of lead on intelligence, their primary centre of interest. Rummo *et al.* (1979) (p. 242) and Albert *et al.* (1974) (p. 243) concluded that there did not appear to be any behavioural deficits in asymptomatic children whereas Kotok *et al.* (1977) (p. 242) came to much the same conclusion when they examined parental ratings of attentional factors.

Baloh *et al.* (1975) (p. 243) continued the pattern of negative results although their measure of behaviour consisted only of an estimate of the children's emotional state while they were being tested.

Conclusions.   The studies in this section do not generally point in the same direction. None was primarily interested in behaviour as an outcome variable and so it could be argued that the measures used lacked sophistication and sensitivity. It must, of course, be remembered that all studies have been criticised on methodological grounds, as outlined in the previous section.

Smelter Studies.   Behavioural results from studies carried out around a known source of lead are easily summed up. Only three attempted to measure behaviour and all came up with negative results.

Lansdown *et al.* (1974) (p. 247) used the Rutter Teachers' Rating Scale and found no association with lead levels and behavioural disturbance, although there was a statistically non-significant association between lead and overactivity.

Also in Britain, Ratcliffe (1977) (p. 248) used a behavioural questionnaire and also found no significant differences, although the trend was for children with higher lead levels to be better behaved.

Finally McNeil *et al.* (1975), working in the El Paso area, used the California Personality Inventory and their results were in line with those found on intelligence tests from the same sample, i.e. no apparent lead effect.

Conclusion.   The conclusion to the section on smelter studies earlier in this chapter was that they are disappointing. In the context of behavioural analysis it is disappointing that so little attention was paid to this topic. The interpretation of the results is qualified by criticisms of study design already dealt with in the previous section.

General Population Studies. As was indicated in the first part of the chapter, these studies came later than most of those already discussed and could therefore address themselves in a more sophisticated way to some of the problem areas thrown up by earlier work. Behavioural difficulties were seen as such a problem by the Lawther Committee who wrote

> ... up to the present no study has satisfactorily demonstrated a relationship between increasing body lead burden and either educational attainment or hyperactivity. Measuring subtle effects requires sophisticated techniques and these have not so far been employed. There are far fewer data on all aspects of behaviour and adjustment other than intelligence. (DHSS, 1980).

One of the studies available to the Lawther Committee was that of Needleman *et al.* (1979) which had used an 11 item forced choice (i.e. the only responses were yes or no) behavioural questionnaire for teachers to rate classroom behaviour on 2146 children. The results were striking for two reasons. In the first place, as Figure 16.1 shows, there was generally a clear dose effect with the higher lead groups doing less well on most items. Secondly, the one item that clearly failed to demonstrate this pattern was, surprisingly, hyperactivity. It must, of course, be noted that these ratings had not been corrected for social factors, a very serious methodological point.

Yule *et al.* (1981) and Lansdown *et al.* (1983) have replicated Needleman's work in their London studies. In the first, pilot study, the results were remarkably similar (Figure 16.2).

The groups were split into four rather than six by lead levels because numbers were too small to do otherwise. But the overall shapes of the histograms were similar, with hyperactivity being noted by very few teachers. As with Needleman, the results were not corrected for social factors.

This study also used the Rutter B(2) Teacher Rating Scale, an instrument of known validity and reliability. The higher 50 per cent of the lead distribution were found to be more often deviant on 20 of the 26 items although statistical significance was reached for only two of them. An examination of the overactivity factor extracted from the Rutter Scale revealed that children with lead levels below 13 μg/100 ml had lower mean activity scores than did

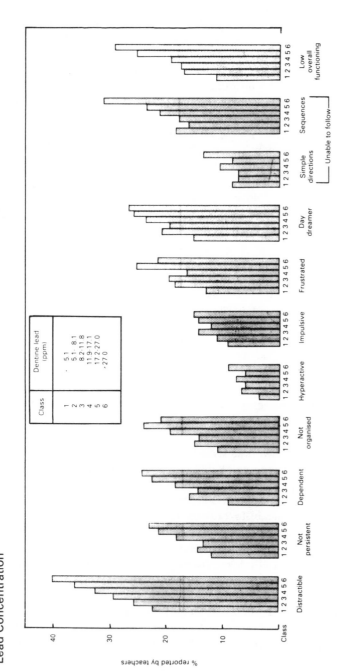

Figure 16.1: Distribution of Negative Ratings by Teachers on 11 Classroom Behaviours in Relation to Dentine Lead Concentration

Source: Needlemann *et al.* (1979)

Figure 16.2: Percentage of Negative Ratings on Needleman Scales by Lead Levels. Pilot lead study — 166 children aged 6-12 years

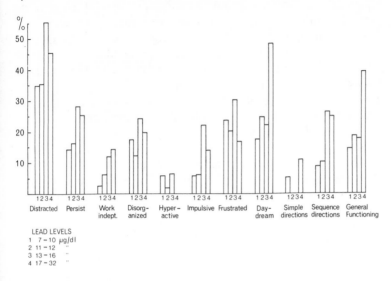

LEAD LEVELS
1 7 – 10 µg/dl
2 11 – 12 "
3 13 – 16 "
4 17 – 32 "

Source: Lansdown *et al.* (1983), p. 275

those with higher levels, statistically significant at the 0.04 level.

A similar picture emerged from the results of the Conner questionnaire, an American measurement which has been widely used in research into hyperactivity. Once more there were indications of a significant association between lead and hyperactivity.

In a discussion on the differences in results the authors point out that Rutter and Conner's scales are more specific than those used by Needleman in their apparent ability to focus attention in a relatively structured classroom learning situation.

Replication is a powerful technique and the parallel findings between the Boston and London Studies was impressive, even if social class had not been considered as a confounding variable. However, the next London study, (Yule *et al.*, 1983) based on children of somewhat different social class, yielded quite different results: there was no association between lead and deviant behaviour even before social class was considered. As was mentioned earlier, the reason for the difference in outcome between the two London studies is far from clear.

Smith *et al.* (1983) included the Conner's Rating Scale in the battery given to their 403 children (discussed on p. 252), and found no evidence of a lead effect either on the total scores or on seven separate factor scores, although there was a tendency for the high lead group to do less well than the low or middle groups.

A somewhat unexpected result came from Milar *et al.* (1981) (see p. 256). The authors used a standardised observation of playroom behaviour as well as two rating scales and found no differences on any measure of hyperactivity even before correcting for social factors. It is not surprising that no lead effect was found, given the other negative results reported in this chapter; what is puzzling is that one would expect differences between the groups on the basis of their home backgrounds alone. It is possible that the tests used were not sufficiently sensitive for the age group studied (over half were less than 3 years old).

Studies of Behaviourally Deviant Children

A leading figure in this field is Oliver David who, with colleagues, has produced a string of studies, mainly focusing on hyperkinesis and lead. David *et al.* (1972) investigated various groups of hyperactive children attending a hospital clinic in New York. Children were classified according to whether they were known to have a 'highly probable cause' of their behaviour (n: 9) a 'possible' cause (n: 8) or were 'pure hyperactive' (n: 54). They were all compared with 37 paediatric clinic controls. If one argues that lead is a powerful factor in hyperactivity then the 'pure hyperactives' would be predicted to have higher lead levels than the other groups.

The 54 'pure hyperactive' children have marginally higher levels than the controls and the 'highly probable cause' group (26.2 vs 22.2 vs 22.9 µg/100 ml). The 'possible cause' group were higher still with a mean of 29.9 µg/100 ml. However, no evidence is available on pica or the social backgrounds of any of the children; the definition of hyperkinesis is not clearly stated and the inter group differences are small.

A subsequent study (David *et al.* 1976) used the same design with larger numbers: 31 'probable cause' children had blood lead levels averaging 20.3 µg/100 ml; 12 'possible cause' had levels averaging 26.3 µg while 41 'aetiology unknown' children averaged 24.7 µg. Combining the 'probable' with the 'possible' groups resulted in a difference of blood lead levels that was not statistically significant. Using results from parental questionnaires no difference was found in the incidence of pica between the groups and there was no information on the sources of lead. This study suffers from similar design weaknesses as are apparent in the former work.

David used a different approach in his 1978 work, presented in a paper to the Conservation Society. He reported correlations between blood lead in 428 children and teachers' ratings on the Conner's Scale. The correlations were, however, very small, being around 0.15. Similar but even lower correlations were found between parent ratings and blood lead levels of 573 children. However, little was reported on the social background and this, plus the fact that data are missing on many children, means that these very small correlations cannot be taken to indicate a causal association.

Chelation Studies

As was mentioned earlier in this chapter the use of chelation promises much theoretically. In behavioural studies it arguably has more to offer than in those concerned with intelligence, since hyperactivity could be expected more readily to respond to changes in assumed causal factors than the more complex constellation making up the functioning assessed by an intelligence test.

Fejerman *et al.* (1973) found that the EEGs and rate of fits changed after chelation in five children with Lennox syndrome. The initial blood leads were not enormously high, 17-40 µg/100 ml, and no information is given on post-chelation levels.

David *et al.* (1976) reported on 13 hyperkinetic children whose original blood lead levels were 25 µg or more. Six had a probable cause ascribed for their hyperkinesis and seven were of unknown aetiology. The former group had lower initial blood lead levels and showed no improvement in behaviour after chelation while the latter seemed, on parent and teacher questionnaires, to have improved. David's conclusion is that this pattern of results implies that lead is a causal factor among those children whose overactivity cannot be explained in other ways. In some ways this is a promising study but the small numbers and the methodological weaknesses noted earlier (p. 246) mean that little can firmly be taken from it.

A much more elaborate design was used by David *et al.*

(1983). Children were deemed to be hyperactive if they were so classified by two of three observers (parent, teacher, doctor) using standardised methods of assessment. A blood lead criterion of 20-50 μg/100 ml was set and children diagnosed as psychotic, mentally or developmentally retarded or as having a significant neurological disease were excluded. As in previous work, three aetiological classifications were used: (a) no known cause; (b) a probable, non-lead related, cause; (c) a history of lead toxicity.

The research design aimed to compare the effects of:

(a) Penicillamine, a chelating agent with no known effect on activity levels.
(b) Methylphenidate, a drug known to reduce inattention/activity but not to affect lead levels.
(c) A placebo.

Children with elevated lead levels without known cause were allocated randomly to one of three treatment regimes:

(1) A comparison of active penicillamine and methylphenidate placebo.
(2) An active methylphenidate and penicillamine placebo.
(3) A comparison of two placebos.

There was, thus, no direct comparison between active penicillamine and active methylphenidate. The design was ABA, i.e. four weeks on the first drug, four on the second and four back on the first. In addition children on the first two regimes received the other placebo throughout.

Almost all children with a history of lead poisoning were assigned to the active penicillamine group but as treatment and evaluation were carried out blind this manipulation of allocation was not seen as invalidating the findings.

The results were:

(1) Active penicillamine was associated with a significant fall in blood lead levels, whereas neither methylphenidate nor the placebo had this effect.
(2) Both active penicillamine and active methylphenidate groups showed significantly improved behaviour when compared to the placebo groups.

(3) There was no significant difference between penicillamine and methylphenidate in their effects on behaviour.

Although this is a far more sophisticated design than David and his co-workers have used before, there are certain reservations to be made about the results. First, despite the blind nature of evaluation, it is unusual to depart from strict randomisation of subjects. Secondly, the lack of a direct comparison of the two active agents is to be regretted. Thirdly, there was a high and variable drop out rate. Fourthly, there is no evidence that behaviour change correlated, within groups, with blood lead reduction. In any case it is unlikely that penicillamine affected brain lead levels (Silbergeld 1983).

Nevertheless, this study is an important contribution to our understanding of the causal effect of lead and stands as an encouragement to the further use of the chelation model.

Conclusions. The classic Byers and Lord (1943) study referred to certain behavioural problems and in a somewhat different context both Patterson (1965) and Bryce-Smith (1971b) raised questions about the effects of lead on behaviour and health. However, even the most recent epidemiological studies have failed to produce convincing *consistent* evidence for an association between moderate levels of lead and behavioural patterns in general; even less is the evidence on lead and hyperactivity. There have been several suggestions and the work on chelation means that the topic should not be dismissed. More than this cannot be said.

References

Albert, R.E., Shore R.E., Sayers, A.J., Strehlow C., Kneip T.J., Pasternak, B.S., Friedhoff, A.J., Coran, F. and Crinono, J.A. (1974) Follow-up of children over exposed to lead. *Environ. Health Perspectives.* 7, 33-9.

Baloh, R., Sturm, R., Green B. and Gleser, B. (1975) Neurophysiological effects of chronic asymptomatic increased lead absorption. *Arch. Neurol., 32*, 326-30.

Beattie, A.D., Moore, M.R., Goldberg, A., Finlayson, M.J.W., Graham, J.F., Mackie, E.M., Main, J.C., McLaren, D.A., Murdoch, R.M. and Stewart, G.T. (1975) Role of chronic low-level lead exposure in the aetiology of mental retardation. *Lancet, i*, 589-92.

Blackman, S.S. (1937) The lesions of lead encephalitis in children. *Bull. Johns Hopkins Hos., 61*, 1-43.

Bornscheim, R., Pearson, D. and Reiter, L. (1980) Behavioural effects of moderate lead exposure in children and animal models. *ILZRO Topical Reviews on Environmental Health Lead 1* International Lead Zinc Organisation, New York.

Bryce-Smith, D. (1971a) Lead pollution — a growing hazard to public health. *Chemistry in Britain, 7,* 54-6.

—— (1971b) Lead pollution from petrol. *Chemistry in Britain, 7,* 284-6.

—— (1972) Behavioural effects of lead and other heavy metal pollutants. *Chemistry in Britain, 8,* 240-3.

—— and Waldron, H.A. (1974) Lead behaviour and criminality. *The Ecologist, 4,* 367-77.

Byers, R.K. and Lord, E.E. (1943) Late effects of lead poisoning on mental development. *Am. J. Dis. Child., 66,* 471-94.

Caldwell, B.M. and Bradley, R.H. (1978) *Administration Manual for the Home Observation for Measurement of the Environment.* University of Arkansas at Little Rock, Arkansas.

Dana, S.L. (1848) *Lead Diseases.* Daniel Bixby, Lowell.

Danielson, L. (1970) *Bulletin No. 6. Ecological Research Committee.* Swedish Natural Science Research Council, Stockholm.

David, O.J., Clark, J. and Voeller, K. (1972) Lead and hyperactivity. *Lancet, ii,* 900-3.

——, Hoffman, S., Clark, J., Grad, G. and Sverd, J. (1983) Penicillamine in the treatment of hyperactive children with moderately elevated lead levels, in M. Rutter and R. Russell Jones (eds.) *Lead Versus Health: The Sources and Effects of Low Level Lead Exposure.* Wiley, Chichester.

——, ——, McCann, b., Sverd, J. and Clark, J. (1976) Low lead levels and mental retardation. *Lancet, ii,* 1376-9.

De la Burdé, B. and Choate, M.S. (1972) Does asymptomatic lead exposure in children have latent sequelae. *J. Pediat., 81,* 1088-91.

—— and —— (1975) Early asymptomatic lead exposure and developmental school age. *J. Pediat., 87,* 638-42.

—— and Shapiro, I.M. (1975) Dental lead, blood lead and pica in urban children. *Arch. Environ. Health, 30,* 281-4.

Elwood, P.C., Morton, M. and St. Leger, A.S. (1976) Lead in water and mental retardation. *Lancet, i,* 590-1.

Ernhart, C.B., Landa, B. and Schell, N.B. (1981) Subclinical levels of lead and developmental deficit — a multivariate follow-up reassessment. *Pediatrics, 67,* 911-19.

Fejerman, N., Gimenez, E.R., Vallego, N.E. and Medina, C.S. (1973) Lennox's syndrome and lead intoxication. *Pediatrics, 52,* 227-34.

Gibson, S.L.M., Larn, C.N., McCrae, W.M. and Goldberg, A. (1967) Blood lead levels in normal and mentally deficient children. *Arch. Dis. Child., 42,* 573-8.

Gregory, R.J., Lehman, R.E. and Mohan, P.J. (1976) Intelligence test results for children with and without undue lead absorption, in G. Wegner (ed.) *Shoshone Lead Health Project.* Idaho Dept. of Health and Welfare.

Harvey, P., Hamlin, M. and Kumar, R. (1983) *The Birmingham Blood Lead Study.* Paper given at the Annual Conference of the British Psychological Society, York, 10th April.

Hebel, J.R., Kinch, D. and Armstrong, E. (1976) Mental capability of children exposed to lead pollution. *Br. J. Prevent. Soc. Med., 30,* 170-4.

Kirkconnell, S.C. and Hicks, L.E. (1980) Residual effects of lead poisoning on Denver Developmental Screening Test scores. *J. Abnormal Child Psychol., 8,* 257-67.

Kotok, D. (1972) Development of children with elevated blood levels: a controlled study. *J. Pediat., 80,* 57-61.

——, Kotok, R. and Heriot, T. (1977) Cognitive Evaluation of children with elevated blood lead levels. *Am. J. Dis. Child., 131,* 791-3.
Landrigan, P.J., Gehlback, S.H., Rosenblum, B.F., Shoulta, J.M., Candelaria, R.M., Bethel, W.F., Liddle, J.A., Smrek, A.L., Staehling, N.M. and Sander, J.D.F. (1975a) Epidemic lead absorption near an ore smelter: the role of particulate lead. *N. Engl. J. Med., 292,* 123-9.
——, Whitworth, R.H., Baloh, R.W., Staehling, M.W., Barthel, W.F. and Rosenblum, B.F. (1975b) Neuropsychological dysfunction in children with chronic low-level lead absorption. *Lancet. i,* 708-12.
Lansdown, R. (1977) *Moderately Raised Lead Levels in Children.* Paper read at a meeting of the Royal Society.
——, Shepherd, J., Clayton, B.E., Delves, H.T., Graham, P.J. and Turner, W.C. (1974) Blood lead levels, behaviour and intelligence: a population study. *Lancet. i,* 538-41.
——, Yule, W., Urbanowicz, M-A. and Millar, I.B. (1983) Blood lead, intelligence attainment and behaviour in school children: overview of a pilot study, in M. Rutter and R. Russell Jones (eds.) *Lead Versus Health: Sources and Effects of Low Level Lead Exposure.* Wiley, Chichester.
McBride, W.G., Black, B.P. and English, B.J. (1982) Blood lead levels and behaviour of 400 preschool children. *Med. J. Aust., 2,* 26-9.
McNeil, J.L., Ptasrik, J.S. and Croft, D.B. (1975) Evaluation of long-term effects of elevated blood lead concentrations in asymptomatic children. *Arch. Ind. Hyg. Toxicol., 26,* (suppl.) 97-118.
Marshall, E. (1983) EPA Faults Classic Lead Poisoning Study. *Science, 222,* 906-7.
Milar, C.B., Schroeder, S.R., Mushak, P. and Boone, L. (1981) Failure to find hyperactivity in preschool children with moderately elevated lead burden. *J. Pediat. Psychol., 6,* 85-95.
Moncrieff, A.A., Konmides, O.P., Clayton, B.E., Patrick, A.D., Rennick, A.G.C. and Roberts, G.C. (1964) Lead poisoning in children. *Arch. Dis. Child., 39,* 1-13.
Moore, M.R., Meredith, P.A. and Goldberg, A. (1977) A retrospective analysis of blood lead in mentally retarded children. *Lancet, i,* 717-19.
Needleman, H.L. (1977) *Studies in Subclinical Lead Exposure. Environmental Health Effects Research Series,* June. Health Effects Research Laboratories, US Environmental Protection Agency, North Carolina.
——, Gunnoe, C., Leviton, A., Reed, M., Peresie, H., Maher, C. and Barrett, P. (1979) Deficits in psychological and classroom performance of children with elevated dentine lead levels. *N. Engl. J. Med., 300,* 689-95.
——, Leviton, A. and Bellinger, D. (1982) Lead-associated intellectual deficit. *N. Engl. J. Med., 306,* 367.
Patterson, C.C. (1965) Contaminated and natural lead environments of man. *Arch. Environ. Health, 11,* 344-60.
Perino, J. and Ernhart, C.B. (1974) The relation of subclinical lead level to cognitive and sensorimotor impairment in black preschoolers. *J. Learning Disorders, 7,* 26-30.
Perlstein, M.A. and Attala, R. (1966) Neurologic sequelae of plumbism in children. *Clin. Pediat., 5,* 292-8.
Pihl, R.D. and Parkes, M. (1977) Hair element content in learning disabled children. *Science, 198,* 204-6.
Pueschel, S.M., Kopito, L. and Schwachman, H. (1972) Children with increased lead burden. *J. Am. Med. Assoc., 222,* 462-6.
Ratcliffe, J.M. (1977) Developmental and behavioural functions in young children with elevated blood lead levels. *Br. J. Preven. Soc. Med., 31,* 258-64.

Rummo, J.H. (1974) *Intellectual and Behavioural Effects of Lead Poisoning in Children.* PhD thesis: University of North Carolina at Chapel Hill.

——, Routh, D.K., Rummo, N.J. and Brown, J.F. (1979) Behavioural and neurological effects of symptomatic and asymptomatic lead exposure in children. *Arch. Environ. Health, 34,* 120-4.

Rutter, M. (1980) Raised lead levels and impaired cognitive/behavioural functioning: A review of the evidence. *Dev. Med. Child Neurol., 22,* Suppl. 42.

Sachs, H.K., Krall, V. and Drayton, M.A. (1982) Neuropsychology assessment after lead poisoning without encephalopathy. *Perceptual Motor Skills, 54,* 1283-8.

——, Krall, V., McCaughran, D.A., Rosenfeld, I.H., Youngsmith, N., Growe, G., Lazar, B., Novar, L., O'Connell, L. and Rayson, B. (1978) I.Q. following treatment of lead poisoning: a patient-sibling comparison. *J. Pediat., 93,* 428-31.

Silbergeld, E.K. (1983) Experimental studies of lead neurotoxicity: Implications for mechanisms, dose response and reversibility, in M. Rutter and R. Russell Jones (eds.) *Lead Versus Health: Sources and Effects of Low Level Lead Exposure.* Wiley, Chichester.

Smith, H.D., Baehner, H.L., Carney, T. and Majors, W.J. (1963) The sequelae of Pica with and without lead poisoning. A comparison of the sequelae five or more years later. *Am. J. Dis. Child, 105,* 609-16.

Smith, M., Delves, T., Lansdown, R., Clayton, B. and Graham, P. (1983) The effects of lead exposure on urban children: the Institute of Child Health/Southampton Study. *Dev. Med. Child Neurol., 25,* Suppl. 47.

Thatcher, R.W., Lester, M.L., McAlaster, R. and Horst, R. (1982) Effects of low levels of cadmium and lead on cognitive functioning in children. *Arch. Environ. Health, 37,* 159-66.

Thomas, H.M. and Blackfan, A.D. (1914) Recurrent meningitis due to lead, in a child of five years. *J. Dis. child., 8,* 377-80.

Wegner, G. (ed.) (1976) *Shoshone Lead Health Project.* Idaho Dept. of Health and Welfare.

Winneke, G., Hrdina, K-G. and Brockhaus, A. (1982) Neuropsychological studies in children with elevated tooth-lead concentrations I. Pilot study. *Int. Arch. Occup. Environ. Health, 51,* 169-83.

——, and Kramer U. (1983) Neuropsychological effects of inorganic lead in children, in K. Blum and L. Manzo (eds.) *Neurotoxicology.* Marcel Dekker, New York.

——, ——, Brockhaus, U., Ewers, U., Kujanek, G., Lechner, H. and Janke, W. (1983) Neuropsychological studies in children with elevated tooth-lead concentrations. II. Extended study. *Int. Arch. Occup. Environ. Health, 51,* 231-52.

Yamin, J. (1976) *The Relationship of Subclinical Lead Intoxication to Cognitive and Language Functioning in Preschool Children.* PhD thesis: Hofstra University.

Yule, W., Lansdown, R., Hunter, J., Urbanowicz, M-A., Clayton, B. and Delves, T. (1983) *Blood Lead Concentrations in School Age Children: Intelligence, Attainment and Behaviour.* Paper given at the Annual Conference of the British Psychological Society.

——, ——, Millar, I.B. and Urbanowicz, M-A. (1981) The relationship between blood lead concentrations, intelligence and attainment in a school population: a pilot study. *Dev. Med. Child Neurol., 23,* 567-76.

Yule, W. and Rutter, M. (1985) Effects of lead on children's behaviour and cognitive performance: a critical review, in K.R. Mahaffey (ed.) *Dietary and Environmental Lead: Human Health Effects.* Elsevier, Amsterdam.

17 CONCLUSIONS

William Yule and Richard Lansdown

In this book, we have had to present the evidence on the effects of lead on children's development in such a way that complicated arguments are more readily understandable by as many readers as possible. Once stripped of scientific jargon and obscurantism, most of the arguments are fairly simple. As the various chapters have demonstrated, the amount of hard evidence on which conclusions have to be based is limited. So why has it been so difficult for campaigners, scientists and governments to reach agreement on whether or not lead at low levels presents a hazard to the health and well-being of our children?

Indeed, we could ask why lead has been the focus of such emotional debate, as opposed to other heavy metals, such as cadmium or zinc, other man-made toxins such as formaldehyde, or other potential environmental health hazards such as noise, radiation, or microwaves? Only time will tell, but we can make some educated guesses. First, the last quarter of the twentieth century has witnessed the parallel growth of consumerism and environmental/ecological awareness, at least within the western democracies. Rightly, one of the concerns of such groups of campaigners has been the effects of industrial and other activity on our environment and on ourselves. Secondly, as we have argued earlier in this book, the effects of high levels of lead exposure being well established it was a plausible hypothesis that lower levels of exposure might have more subtle effects on behaviours. Thirdly, and tellingly, the possible effects on children were publicised, and these have more emotional appeal than the effects on working people at their work place. Fourthly, having (rightly or wrongly) identified lead in petrol as a major culprit, there seemed to be an easy solution on which to focus a campaign. Fifthly, given the conflicting interests of multinational companies, governments and 'innocent children', all the ingredients were present for good editorial copy about cover-ups. So far, none of the other health hazards have this combination of factors operating simultaneously.

Whatever the causes, the imagination and emotion of the public was soon fired. Lead, especially in petrol, was known to be guilty

of doing untold damage to children. Governments had to act —
and they did so in the time-honoured tradition of asking for
reports from experts. When expert committees did not produce
simple recommendations in line with public opinion, charges of
bias and cover-up abounded.

From our point of view as members of the Lawther committee,
nothing in our previous training or experience had prepared us for
the experience of trying to evaluate scientific evidence against the
background of populist pressure and in some cases, personal
attack. During the debates in the press, scientific and political
judgements were often confused. Scientists take pride in seeing all
sides of the argument; journalists want to communicate simple
conclusions devoid of caveats (and to sell papers through eye-
catching headlines). Politicians have to take policy decisions.

Careful reading of the Lawther Report (DHSS, 1980) will show
that all of the issues raised in this book were considered and,
contrary to the misrepresentations following its publication, the
Report concluded that although the evidence of the effects of low
levels of lead exposure on children's health was meagre, nevertheless lead from all sources should be reduced. The Report went
as far as to say:

> Emissions of lead to the air from traffic and other sources
> should be progressively reduced, subject to an appraisal of any
> other possible effects on health of altering the constituents of
> petrol ... (DHSS, 1980: paragraph 5, p. 52)

and all people familiar with simple mathematics (but few journalists or campaigners) realise that 'progressive reduction' from a
finite starting point can only end in zero. The *rate* at which lead
should be reduced from petrol was seen as a political rather than a
scientific question.

Since the publication of the Lawther Report, various governments have taken action to reduce lead in the environment —
especially from paint and petrol. The publication of the Ninth
Report of the Royal Commission on Environmental Pollution
(1983) served to complete the arguments. They concluded,

> 8.19. At present the average blood lead concentration of the
> UK population is about one quarter of that at which features of
> frank lead poisoning may occasionally occur. We are not aware

of any other toxin which is so widely distributed in human and animal populations and which is also universally present at levels that exceed even one tenth of that at which clinical signs and symptoms may occur ...

8.20 ... In our view it would be prudent to take steps to increase the safety margin for the population as a whole. We reach this conclusion without coming to any judgement on the possible effects of low concentration of lead on children's behaviour ...

8.21. We conclude that measures should be taken to reduce the anthropogenic dispersal of lead wherever possible ... (Royal Commission on Environmental Pollution, 1983)

At least, the political arguments were over — the scientific questions remained open or in the old Scots verdict, 'not proven'.

This book has presented a review of the evidence, concentrating on the most recent studies published since 1979. Recently, the Medical Research Council has produced the report of a small, expert committee which also reviews this evidence and concluded:

In Summary, the evidence most appropriate to British children comes from recent findings by three research teams, Smith *et al.*, Yule *et al.*, and Harvey *et al.* All three found no statistically significant association between body lead burden and IQ after allowance for compounding factors. Because of the nature of cross-sectional population surveys, one can never demonstrate conclusively that there is *no* effect. However, the available evidence suggests that a considerable elevation in body lead burden, as found in some British children, has little or no effect on IQ (MRC, 1984: Paragraph 5.15, p. 19: emphasis in original).

In our view there are two broad conclusions to the lead debate. The first is one restricted to a scientific interpretation of data from research studies. As scientists we accept the MRC conclusions as far as they go. But we note that they do not say that low levels of lead have no effect, only that available evidence on British children suggests that a moderate elevation has little or no effect. In other words, there remains a possibility that the effect is greater, or more complex, or more subtle, than has hitherto been shown.

Support for caution is provided by preliminary results from a population study of over 570 11-year olds living in Dunedin, New Zealand (Silva *et al.*, 1984). Their average blood lead level was 11.1 µg/100 ml, some 2 µg/100 ml lower than our London sample. Despite this, and despite the older, homogeneous age range, significant relationships were found with academic attainment and behaviour, with near-significant relationships with verbal IQ, in a situation in which the children's levels were *not* related to socioeconomic status. These results add to the growing body of evidence that low levels of lead exposure do have effects on children's development.

Nor do we dismiss the notion that a possible effect is differential in its manifestation; that is, it may appear more strongly in children who are also disadvantaged in other ways. If this is so, then even more complexity is added to the task of weighing evidence.

The second conclusion is related to action. If there remains the possibility of an effect of lead on children's development it would be prudent to take whatever steps are necessary to remove it from the environment. At least it is easier to control the emission of lead from several sources than it is to improve attainment and adjustment through education at home and at school.

Even these conclusions may have to be modified once the exact mode of action of lead on the central nervous system is better understood. As the chapters on animal studies, intelligence and behaviour have all emphasised, until there are better models of action of lead on the CNS, it is difficult to know which functions of behaviour to measure. Existing tests of neuropsychological functioning are very crude and as they improve, so more specific relationships may become clearer.

From a scientific point of view the studies reviewed in this book raise fundamental questions about the relationships between brain and behaviour. All behaviour is the outcome of interactions between genetic influences, subsequent social experience, diet and a myriad of other environmental factors. Given that intelligence and adjustment are the outcome of the interplay of so many factors, it is not surprising that it has proven difficult to isolate the effect of just one bearing on children's functioning. And yet the work of the past decade has highlighted the methodological problems involved and the need to develop new, more sensitive measures of specific functions such as attention, learning and memory.

All of the problems encountered in investigating lead are present in investigating the effects of other environmental pollutants and toxins. In effect, a new subspecialty of child psychology has been conceived (if not yet born) — what might be termed developmental behavioural toxicology. In part, a case for the extension of the role of psychologists has been argued by Fein *et al.* (1983), especially in relation to the effect of environmental toxins on fetuses *in utero*. What we are arguing is that there is a need to develop greater expertise in monitoring and isolating the effects of various environmental influences on children's development. Many of the techniques of enquiry are well developed in the largely medical subspecialty of epidemiology. What, so far, is missing is a fuller appreciation of the nature and measurement of human, psychological, individual differences. Psychological tests are not like biochemical tests — they are considerably more reactive and dependent on the tester both for administration and scoring. These facts alone make the use of psychological test data more difficult than physiological or biochemical data. Thus, there is a need for much closer interdisciplinary collaboration between child psychologists and other professionals to investigate the effects of toxins on children's development. Many of the basic concepts and much of the technology needed as the basis for such collaborative work already exist. What is now required is the commitment and funding to facilitate the development of the new specialty. Without the development of such expertise, professionals and public alike can only react in piecemeal fashion to investigating newly identified hazards. Combined with national and international programmes of environmental studies, developmental behavioural toxicology can play a vital role in the detection of toxic effects and the prevention of widescale problems.

References

DHSS (1980) *Lead and Health: The Report of a DHSS Working Party on Lead in the Environment* (Chairman: Professor P. Lawther). HMSO, London.

Fein, G.G., Schwartz, P.M., Jacobson, S.W. and Jacobson, J.L. (1983) Environmental toxins and behavioral development: A new role for psychological research. *Am. Psychol., 38*, 1183-97.

Medical Research Council (1984) *The Neuropsychological Effects of Lead in Children: A Review of Recent Research: 1979-1983*. MRC, London.

Royal Commission on Environmental Pollution (1983) *Ninth Report: Lead in the Environment*. HMSO, London.

Silva, P.A., Hughes, P., Crosado, B. and Faed, J. (1984) Preliminary
Communication: A pilot study of blood lead levels, cognitive development, and
behaviour problems in 579 Dunedin Eleven year old children. Paper presented
at Workshop on Lead Research, University of Auckland, New Zealand, 27th
November 1984. University of Otago Medical School, Dunedin.

GLOSSARY

ALA dehydratase the second enzyme of haem biosynthesis

alginates organic substances used in foodstuffs and prepared generally from seaweeds

alkyl halide organic compound which contains one of the three halogen elements: chlorine, bromine or iodine

atomic weight the weight of an atom of an element as compared with that of an element of hydrogen taken as unity: also the sum of the weights of the atoms of a compound

bacterial methylation addition of methyl (alkyl) groups which are organic subcompounds to other organic compounds by bacteria

binding sites positions on biological molecules to which materials may bind

bioavailable a material is bioavailable if some biological system can use it

carboxyl a ligand binding group which is an organic acid containing carbon oxygen (2) and hydrogen

cellular organelles the small particles that make up the interior components of the cell, such as mitochondria

chelating agents drugs or chemicals which can bind ions like lead and make them more soluble. They can be used to reduce lead concentrations in an organism.

cholecalciferol supplementation added vitamin D

cilia the small, hair like structure on the cell wall of absorptive cells

cytochrome P 450 a mono-oxygenase group of enzymes used to oxidise drugs and foreign chemicals

desquamation the breaking away of cells from a surface as is found in the skin

duplicate diet exactly the same meals and drinks that a person consumes, taken separately for analysis

ecosystems a system which involves the interaction of the living community with its non-living environment

erythrocyte the red cell of the blood

ethanol ethyl alcohol or alcohol

eutetic melting readily

haem an iron protoporphyrin compound which constitutes the pigment portion of the haemoglobin molecule and is responsible for its oxygen-carrying properties

haematocrit the volume percentage of red blood cells in whole blood

haemoglobin the oxygen carrying pigment of the red blood cells, made up of four haem molecules bound to four globin polypeptide chains

half-life the time taken for half of the amount of lead (or other substances) to be lost from the system

hypertransfusion greater than normal transfusion

in vitro a biological process occurring outside a living organism in an artificial environment

inverted intestinal sack preparations the intestine turned inside out

ionic lead lead in a soluble form bound to other ions such as chloride

jejunal relating to part of the small intestine

kinetic models a system made of mathematical equations which approximates to the reaction of lead in the body

lead aerosols extremely small particles of lead suspended in the air

ligand binding means by which chemical groups, for example proteins, can link to other compounds

lipids fats

lumen of the gastrointestinal tract the inside of the small intestine

matrix interference the way in which the structure of the analytical system interferes with the signal produced by lead

organic applied to a class of compound substances which naturally exist as constituents of organised bodies or are formed from compounds which so exist. Thus organic lead compounds are those which contain carbon, hydrogen and oxygen.

protoporphyrin the last compound of haem biosynthesis. This is the compound into which iron is inserted to make up haem.

radionuclide for skeletal imaging radioactive compound which is taken up preferentially by bone

ribosomes one of the cellular organelles which contain nucleic acids (genetic material)

rumen digestion the type of digestion used by ruminant animals such as the cow

serosal relating to the serous membrane

serum levels of 1,25 dihydroxy vitamin D levels of one component (the active one) of vitamin D in the blood serum (not red cells)

sulphydryl a ligand binding group which comprises sulphur and hydrogen

trophic related to nutrition or feeding

tubular reabsorption a function of the kidney

ultrastructural autoradiography the visualisation of the structure of a cell by uptake of radioactive materials and their printing on photographic film

venturi the narrowing of a tube which increases the speed of a fluid flowing through that tube

wet ashing the destruction of organic compounds by chemicals, usually strong acids

APPENDIX

Conversion table from μmoles/litre to μg/100 ml

μmol/litre	μg/100 ml
0.1	2.07
0.2	4.14
0.3	6.21
0.4	8.28
0.5	10.35
0.6	12.42
0.7	14.49
0.8	16.56
0.9	18.63
1.0	20.70
2.0	41.40
3.0	62.11
4.0	82.81
5.0	103.51
6.0	124.22
7.0	144.93
8.0	165.63
9.0	186.33
10.0	207.03

INDEX